D0876867

Robert G. Anderson, ThM
Mary A. Fukuyama, PhD
Editors

Ministry in the Spiritual and Cultural Diversity of Health Care: Increasing the Competency of Chaplains

Ministry in the Spiritual and Cultural Diversity of Health Care: Increasing the Competency of Chaplains has been co-published simultaneously as *Journal of Health Care Chaplaincy,* Volume 13, Number 2 2004.

*Pre-publication
REVIEWS,
COMMENTARIES,
EVALUATIONS . . .*

"**E**SPECIALLY WORTHWHILE....
Equips chaplains to develop ongoing competency as educators and practitioners in cultural and spiritual diversity both within and beyond their health care settings. As a health care chaplain and as Chair of our health care system's Transcultural Strategic Task Force, I appreciate this challenging book for two reasons. One, it's addressed specifically to meet the needs of chaplains; and two, the emphasis is on increasing our competency."

Richard M. Leliaert, PhD
Manager, Spiritual Support Services and Chair, Transcultural Strategic Taskforce, Oakwood Hospital and Medical Center, Dearborn, Michigan

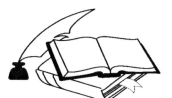

The Haworth Pastoral Press
An Imprint of The Haworth Press, Inc.

Ministry in the Spiritual and Cultural Diversity of Health Care: Increasing the Competency of Chaplains

Ministry in the Spiritual and Cultural Diversity of *Health Care: Increasing the Competency of Chaplains* has been co-published simultaneously as *Journal of Health Care Chaplaincy*, Volume 13, Number 2 2004.

The *Journal of Health Care Chaplaincy* Monographic "Separates"

Below is a list of "separates," which in serials librarianship means a special issue simultaneously published as a special journal issue or double-issue *and* as a "separate" hardbound monograph. (This is a format which we also call a "DocuSerial.")

"Separates" are published because specialized libraries or professionals may wish to purchase a specific thematic issue by itself in a format which can be separately cataloged and shelved, as opposed to purchasing the journal on an on-going basis. Faculty members may also more easily consider a "separate" for classroom adoption.

"Separates" are carefully classified separately with the major book jobbers so that the journal tie-in can be noted on new book order slips to avoid duplicate purchasing.

You may wish to visit Haworth's website at . . .

http://www.HaworthPress.com

. . . to search our online catalog for complete tables of contents of these separates and related publications.

You may also call 1-800-HAWORTH (outside US/Canada: 607-722-5857), or Fax 1-800-895-0582 (outside US/Canada: 607-771-0012), or e-mail at:

docdelivery@haworthpress.com

Ministry in the Spiritual and Cultural Diversity of Health Care: Increasing the Competency of Chaplains, edited by Robert G. Anderson, ThM, and Mary A. Fukuyama, PhD (Vol. 13, No. 2, 2004). *"All clergy and health care professionals interested in the spiritual dimensions of cultual competence will want to read this book. Discussions of cultural competence too often neglect the spiritual dimensions. This book fills that gap." (Rev. John R. deVelder, DMin, Convener, International Network ACPE; Vice Chair, Congress in Ministry in Specialized Settings Network (COMTSS Network); Director, Pastoral Care Department, Robert Wood Johnson University Hospital).*

Professional Chaplaincy and Clinical Pastoral Education Should Become More Scientific: Yes and No. edited by Larry VandeCreek, DMin, BCC (Vol. 12, No. 1/2, and Vol. 13, No. 1, 2002). *"Timely. . . . Must reading for anyone concerned about the future of chaplaincy in health care settings and about the relationship of spirituality, religion, and health." (Augustine Meier, PhD, Professor Emeritus, Clinical Psychology, Saint Paul University)*

The Discipline for Pastoral Care Giving: Foundations for Outcome Oriented Chaplaincy, edited by Larry VandeCreek, DMin, BCC, and Arthur M. Lucas, MDiv, BCC (Vol. 10, No. 2, 2001 and Vol. 11, No. 1, 2001). *"A cutting edge approach to spiritual care. . . . An essential resource." (George Fitchett, DMin, Associate Professor and Director of Research, Rush-Presbyterian-St. Luke's Medical Center, Chicago, Illinois)*

Professional Chaplaincy: What Is Happening to It During Health Care Reform? edited by Larry VandeCreek, DMin, BCC (Vol. 10, No. 1, 2000). *Containing firsthand accounts of the present changes in the field and suggestions for action from an Australian case study, this informative work will assist you in developing future plans for chaplaincy, ones that will take your needs into consideration and help this important job remain in care facilities.*

Contract Pastoral Care and Education: The Trend of the Future? edited by Larry VandeCreek, DMin, BCC (Vol. 9, No. 1/2, 1999). *Provides clergy of all faiths and students with information on how religious and spiritual ministries within health care benefit patients. You will discover "how to" suggestions as well as a wealth of experiences and models for planning a freestanding pastoral care center of your own to benefit your community.*

Spiritual Care for Persons with Dementia: Fundamentals for Pastoral Practice, edited by Larry VandeCreek, DMin, BCC (Vol. 8, No. 1/2, 1999). *Offers you a better understanding of dementia and how to better serve persons with this frustrating and often confusing disease.*

Scientific and Pastoral Perspectives on Intercessory Prayer: An Exchange Between Larry Dossey, MD and Health Care Chaplains, edited by Larry VandeCreek, DMin (Vol. 7, No. 1/2, 1998). *"Anyone who wonders about our prayers and our needs will be drawn into these dialogues." (Laland E. Elhard, PhD, Professor of Pastoral Theology, Trinity Lutheran Seminary, Columbus, Ohio) Summarizes Larry Dossey's work on prayer and challenges chaplains to think seriously about its role in their ministry.*

Ministry of Hospital Chaplains: Patient Satisfaction, edited by Larry VandeCreek, DMin, and Marjorie A. Lyon (Vol. 6, No. 2, 1997). *Explores patient satisfaction with the general hospital chaplain's ministry.*

Organ Transplantation in Religious, Ethical, and Social Context: No Room for Death, edited by William R. DeLong, MDiv, FCOC (Vol. 5, No. 1/2, 1993). *"I recommend this book to anyone working with transplant recipients or donor families." (Sharon Augustine, RN, MS, Heart and Lung Transplant Service, The Johns Hopkins Hospital, Baltimore)*

Health Care Chaplaincy in Oncology, edited by Laurel Arthur Burton, ThD, and George Handzo, MDiv (Vol. 4, No. 1/2, 1993). *"A valuable collection that speaks of the 'Modern' professional chaplain." (Rev. Elaine Hickman, Manager, Chaplaincy Services, Mercy General Hospital; President, The College of Chaplains, Inc.; Vice President, COMISS (Congress on Ministry in Specialized Settings))*

The Chaplain-Physician Relationship, edited by Larry VandeCreek, DMin, and Laurel Arthur Burton, ThD (Vol. 3, No. 2, 1993). *"Recommended to both chaplains and physicians who are searching for ways to overcome the relational distance between the two professions." (The Journal of Pastoral Care)*

Making Chaplaincy Work: Practical Approaches, edited by Laurel Arthur Burton, ThD (Vol. 1, No. 2, 1988). *"Dr. Burton has done a first-class job of bringing together articulate writers whose content has been informed by their daily practice of ministry within healthcare settings." (David E. Latham, Director of Chaplaincy Services, Community United Methodist Hospital, Henderson, Kentucky)*

Published by

The Haworth Pastoral Press, 10 Alice Street, Binghamton, NY 13904-1580 USA

The Haworth Pastoral Press is an imprint of The Haworth Press, Inc., 10 Alice Street, Binghamton, NY 13904-1580 USA.

Ministry in the Spiritual and Cultural Diversity of Health Care: Increasing the Competency of Chaplains has been co-published simultaneously as *Journal of Health Care Chaplaincy,* Volume 13, Number 2 2004.

The development, preparation, and publication of this work has been undertaken with great care. However, the publisher, employees, editors, and agents of The Haworth Press and all imprints of The Haworth Press, Inc., including The Haworth Medical Press® and The Pharmaceutical Products Press®, are not responsible for any errors contained herein or for consequences that may ensue from use of materials or information contained in this work. Opinions expressed by the author(s) are not necessarily those of The Haworth Press, Inc.

Cover design by Jennifer M. Gaska.

Library of Congress Cataloging-in-Publication Data

Ministry in the spiritual and cultural diversity of health care: increasing the competency of chaplains/ Robert G. Anderson and Mary A. Fukuyama, editors.
    p. cm.
    "Ministry in the spiritual and cultural diversity of health care co-published simultaneously as Journal of Heath Care Chaplaincy, volume 13, number 2 2004."
    Includes bibliographical references and index.
    ISBN 0-7890-2556-6 (hard cover: alk. paper)-ISBN 0-7890-2557-4) (soft cover: alk. paper)
1. Chaplains, Hospital. 2. Religious pluralism. 3. Pluralism (Social sciences) I. Anderson, Robert G.
II Fukuyama, Mary A. III. Journal of health care chaplaincy.

BV4335.M55 2004
259'.411–'dc22   2004014036

Ministry in the Spiritual and Cultural Diversity of Health Care: Increasing the Competency of Chaplains

Robert G. Anderson, ThM
Mary A. Fukuyama, PhD
Editors

Ministry in the Spiritual and Cultural Diversity of Health Care: Increasing the Competency of Chaplains has been co-published simultaneously as *Journal of Health Care Chaplaincy*, Volume 13, Number 2 2004.

The Haworth Pastoral Press®
An Imprint of The Haworth Press, Inc.

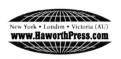

New York • London • Victoria (AU)
www.HaworthPress.com

133194

Indexing, Abstracting & Website/Internet Coverage

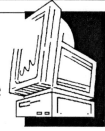

This section provides you with a list of major indexing & abstracting services. That is to say, each service began covering this periodical during the year noted in the right column. Most Websites which are listed below have indicated that they will either post, disseminate, compile, archive, cite or alert their own Website users with research-based content from this work. (This list is as current as the copyright date of this publication.)

Abstracting, Website/Indexing Coverage . . . . Year When Coverage Began

- *ATLA Religion Database with ATLASerials. This periodical is indexed in ATLA Religion Database with ATLASerials, published by the American Theological Library Association <http://atla.com>.* **1988**
- *This periodical is indexed in ATLA Religion Database, published by the American Theological Library Association <http://www.atla.com>* . . . . *
- *AURSI African Urban & Regional Science Index. A scholarly & research index which synthsises & compiles all pubilcations on urbanization & regional science in Africa within the world. Published annually* **2004**
- *CINAHL (Cumulative Index to Nursing & Allied Health Literature), in print, EBSCO, and SilverPlatter, DataStar, and PaperChase. (Support materials include Subject Heading List, Database Search Guide, and instructional video) <http://cinahl.com>* **2000**
- *Current Thoughts & Trends "Abstracts Section" <http://CurrentThoughts.com>* **2000**
- *Family & Society Studies Worldwide <http://www.nisc.com>* **1995**
- *Family Index Database <http://www.familyscholar.com>* **2004**

(continued)

   *Exact start date to come.

Special Bibliographic Notes related to special journal issues (separates) and indexing/abstracting:

- indexing/abstracting services in this list will also cover material in any "separate" that is co-published simultaneously with Haworth's special thematic journal issue or DocuSerial. Indexing/abstracting usually covers material at the article/chapter level.
- monographic co-editions are intended for either non-subscribers or libraries which intend to purchase a second copy for their circulating collections.
- monographic co-editions are reported to all jobbers/wholesalers/approval plans. The source journal is listed as the "series" to assist the prevention of duplicate purchasing in the same manner utilized for books-in-series.
- to facilitate user/access services all indexing/abstracting services are encouraged to utilize the co-indexing entry note indicated at the bottom of the first page of each article/chapter/contribution.
- this is intended to assist a library user of any reference tool (whether print, electronic, online, or CD-ROM) to locate the monographic version if the library has purchased this version but not a subscription to the source journal.
- individual articles/chapters in any Haworth publication are also available through the Haworth Document Delivery Service (HDDS).

Ministry in the Spiritual and Cultural Diversity of Health Care: Increasing the Competency of Chaplains

CONTENTS

ABOUT THE EDITORS

Robert G. Anderson, ThM, is the Clinical Pastoral Education Supervisor and Chaplain of the Department of Pastoral Care and Education at the New York Presbyterian Hospital. He has served as an ACPE chaplain supervisor and staff chaplain in four metropolitan hospital settings over the past 32 years. Through relationships with patients, their families and loved ones, and with medical and hospital staff, he has come to recognize the necessity and exhilaration of learning and growing with spiritual and cultural diversity.

Mary A. Fukuyama, PhD, is a Clinical Professor and Counseling Psychologist at the University of Florida in Gainesville. Mary's professional interests include Multicultural Counseling and training, Asian-American concerns, multiple identities, and spiritual issues in counseling. She recently published a book titled *Integrating Spirituality into Multicultural Counseling* with Todd Sevig from the University of Michigan. She continues to seek ways in which multiculturalism can be infused into counseling and training. Her theoretical orientation is humanistic-existential, and she enjoys Gestalt therapy and dream work.

The Search for Spiritual/
Cultural Competency
in Chaplaincy Practice:
Five Steps that Mark the Path

Robert G. Anderson, ThM

SUMMARY. Chaplains who are clinically trained and certified spiritual care professionals can make a unique contribution in today's increasingly pluralistic and global health care context with diverse religious, spiritual and cultural values, beliefs and practices. The author characterizes this contribution as spiritual/cultural competency. A self-defined web of meaning is unique to each person, comprised of a composite of values and beliefs, a fabric woven by way of one's life narrative. The proven approach of clinical learning, with heightened introspective and interpersonal awareness, serves as the chaplain's primary pathway to multi-spiritual/cultural competency, integrated with the exploration of context in a way not prioritized before. Utilizing sources

---

Robert G. Anderson is affiliated with New York Presbyterian Hospital, Weill Cornell Medical Center, New York, NY (E-mail: rga9001@nyp.org).

[Haworth co-indexing entry note]: "The Search for Spiritual/Cultural Competency in Chaplaincy Practice: Five Steps that Mark the Path." Anderson, Robert G. Co-published simultaneously in *Journal of Health Care Chaplaincy* (The Haworth Pastoral Press, an imprint of The Haworth Press, Inc.) Vol. 13, No. 2, 2004, pp. 1-24; and: *Ministry in the Spiritual and Cultural Diversity of Health Care: Increasing the Competency of Chaplains* (ed: Robert G. Anderson, and Mary A. Fukuyama) The Haworth Pastoral Press, an imprint of The Haworth Press, Inc., 2004, pp. 1-24. Single or multiple copies of this article are available for a fee from The Haworth Document Delivery Service [1-800-HAWORTH, 9:00 a.m. - 5:00 p.m. (EST). E-mail address: docdelivery@haworthpress.com].

Digital Object Identifier: 10.1300/J080v13n02_01

from pastoral theology, anthropology and multicultural counseling, a five-step process of competency assessment is introduced and discussed with the aid of two cases. Knowing one's own spiritual/cultural grounding is the first step in this open-ended search. *[Article copies available for a fee from The Haworth Document Delivery Service: 1-800-HAWORTH. E-mail address: <docdelivery@haworthpress.com> Website: <http://www.HaworthPress.com> © 2004 by The Haworth Press, Inc. All rights reserved.]*

KEYWORDS. Multicultural chaplaincy, religion, spirituality

INTRODUCTION

As human communities in North America become more global and diverse, the cultural, religious, and spiritual elements of individual and gathered life are more varied, complex and interwoven. The constellation of diverse faith communities with Muslim beliefs and practices is as complex as that of Protestantism, leading to countless variety. Those who provide spiritual care and counseling in hospital and other settings, especially certified health care chaplains, have a responsibility to develop competencies that respond to the concerns and distresses expressed in uniquely spiritual and cultural ways by the person, family and kin in life transitions and crises. Thornton (1970) describes such professional competency as an ongoing process of mastery, learning, and maturation, combining elements historically developed in the clinical pastoral education movement.

In this article we will explore the challenge for the globalized spiritual care professional in health care to address emotional, cultural and spiritual needs. It is crucial to comprehend the cultural and spiritual characteristics that comprise individual identity and meaning. This personal constellation has been identified as a demographic composite or listing of generalized categories of affiliation, groups or sub-groups to which the person belongs. They are, in fact, internalized elements of identity, unique to every person. An example of that internalization might be, "When I tell you that I am a 45-year-old married Puerto Rican male with three jobs and a critically ill mother in this hospital, you've got the whole picture."

Only the person in transition or crisis can describe the elements that comprise identity and meaning in their life. Assumptions about ethnic, religious, and age groups distort the understanding of a particular person and are often the presumptions of the dominant religious or cultural view regarding those different from the prevailing custom and culture. Surprisingly, the Puerto Rican quoted above, a third generation native of the metropolis where he lives, is tall and blue eyed.

Chaplains providing spiritual care in hospital settings have unexpected challenges. "I'm puzzled by the different people coming to our ER. How do I relate to them? Sometimes they don't speak English. Imagine, the nursing staff is turning to me!" In the chaplain's repertoire is the proven resource of process learning based in clinical pastoral education. That process approach fosters continuous formation in the reflective practice of ministry. To meet the challenge of the pluralistic and globalized health care context, chaplains must first grasp their own spiritual/cultural constellation, what might best be described as a web of meaning, through self-assessment and definition. Second, chaplains need to develop a capacity to assess and understand the spiritual/cultural constellation, the web of meaning of the person with whom they are professionally relating. I have chosen to refer to such a dual professional capacity as "spiritual/cultural competency." Recent literature and expertise developed in complementary fields, especially multicultural counseling, can serve as primary resources in shaping our enterprise.

Soon after the puzzled chaplain describes his ER dilemma, he gets a frantic long distance telephone call from his daughter on a bicycle tour in Thailand. She has broken her leg in a mishap and has to stay in a small hospital while the group travels back to Bangkok. His daughter describes panic at not speaking Thai and bewilderment that staff laughs a lot around her. The chaplain is challenged to weigh and correlate what is out of the range of previous life experience. New awareness emerges out of two chaotic and challenging situations.

A well defined perspective that celebrates and continuously learns from our pluralistic communal context of life and work fosters an open-ended framework for spiritual care practice. The legitimacy of a countless variety of cultural, spiritual, and religious beliefs and practices is recognized, a matrix more pluralistic and complex than a Judeo-Christian framework with embedded assumptions and shared beliefs. What we seek in this article is an open-ended, descriptive and inclusive framework for globalized multi-faith North America, setting guidelines for competence in an open ended and diverse society. This search is a journey without a necessary destination.

THE UNIVERSAL, CULTURAL, AND INDIVIDUAL ELEMENTS OF LIFE NARRATIVE

The boundaries of our societies, cities, neighborhoods, and families are fluid and their composition heterogeneous. Cultural, religious, and spiritual dimensions of life join together to create meaning on a daily basis. A Reform Jewish/Methodist couple adopts a toddler from China, makes their first trip to Asia, studies Buddhism and hires a Chilean Catholic woman, mother of 3, to provide weekday childcare. A third generation Italian Catholic discovers his family name was Jewish until his great grandfather arrived at Ellis Island in 1900. Personal heritage is a feature of migrations, crises, sufferings, and surprises that makes our identity rich and multi-faceted. In the midst of life transition and crisis, aspects of culture, religion, and spirituality comprise core and interrelated components of personal and communal identity. At a recent seminar an anthropologist told a chaplaincy group, "If you look back over a few generations, likely we all were refugees." The ethnic identity of a person shaped in life narrative has a particular meaning, shaped by and unique within a cultural entity that may be attributed to the person as part of a collective group. For our purpose, the individual, more than the group will be the focus as the carrier of culture (Note 1).

Augsburger (1986) has valuably interpreted the work of Kluckhohn and Murray (1948) in describing the universal, cultural, and individual dimensions of humanity. We are biologically similar, eat and drink, have a life span and relate to others, essentials that make us "like all others." We are drawn to and gather with select people, participate in family and group rituals, value and observe life and work in keeping with others, speak a particular language, essentials that make us "like some others." We also have a personality, singular feelings and thoughts, habits and devotions, essentials that are "like no other." The universal, cultural, and individual essentials make up our worldview and all are laden with meaning, the dimension of life that saturates our reality. Geertz (1973) refers to culture as our "web of significance (p. 5)." I see the web as including these three dimensions spun together in a selective way in what I would refer to as a web of meaning. The Reform Jewish/Methodist couple defines a web of meaning centered on the adoption of a Chinese infant within their family and the shaping of a community context to hold diverse elements of their shared beliefs and identity. Meaning is thus shaped by internalized collective and communal elements.

Spiritual care providers often miss this uniquely woven core composite due to a prevailing Christian or even Judeo-Christian understanding of individuality that often coincides in the health care context with a worldview based upon positivistic, linear, and scientific Western thought. Sue (1998) refers to the "invisible veil" of the prevailing culture that blocks comprehension (p. 16). In developing competence one needs to exchange the assumption that reality is shared for the working assumption that reality is not shared. The chaplain's religious, ecumenical or even interfaith perspective, tailored to the hospital's reliance upon the efficacy of acute diagnosis and treatment can combine as a formidable veil, a barrier whereby caregivers overlook the differing worldview of a frightened, disoriented and isolated person and family.

The patient and family struggling to face the juncture of life and death, even with the chaplain's aid, can be confounded by an embedded clash within the hospital between initiatives for aggressive acute care and aggressive comfort care. Such dynamics highlight forces and tensions, aspects of multi-cultural complexity in the organization worthy of attention at another time. I emphasize the personal constellation of the patient's values and beliefs. It is important to acknowledge that the assumptions and values inherent in the hospital context complicate this understanding. The chaplain's essential contribution as an interpreter of spiritual/cultural dynamics requires the use clinical sensitivity, already available to the serious chaplain. Let us seek to broaden and integrate the proven approach of clinical learning with multi-spiritual and cultural awareness.

THE LIVING HUMAN DOCUMENT AND MEANING

Emerging out of North American liberal Anglo Protestant thought of the early 1900s, the clinical pastoral education movement pioneered an exploration of individuals in crisis by acknowledging and utilizing depth psychology and the behavioral sciences through the case study method. Initially, this venture fostered a dialogue in theological and ministerial education about the religious meaning and mystery of the human personality in the context of severe life crisis. Anton Boisen (1953) referred to the person as "a living human document," (p. 3) a source for research so as to learn in depth about the meaning and unique elements of life narrative (Note 2). The clinical setting of the hospital became the primary context to conduct case studies and to explore pastoral relationships, to learn through supervised observation, reflection and interaction about patient-chaplain encounters and effective ways of providing pastoral care and counseling. The focus was primarily upon universal and individual features of human meaning from a depth perspective. Internalized religion was identified with universal and individual features but less for particular cultural dimensions. When culture was acknowledged it was in terms of group identity and custom and not a particularized integrated element.

While this century old movement incorporated religious, moral, social and psychological factors in the assessment of the person, culture was an external force contending with religion in the societal arena. A particular cluster of beliefs, values, and worldviews based upon cultural and spiritual identity did not weigh in as essential in studying the individual in context. I contend that the cultural and spiritual factors when viewed in a more integrated way enrich the life narrative of the living human document and shape unique meaning. Such attitudes, values and beliefs carried into the life crisis are just as primary as psychological and developmental features to explain and interpret life journey, the surprises, sorrows, and joys that comprise life narrative, and the life juncture one faces, the unfolding chapter of the present.

Defining culture, spirituality and religion would be important for our discussion. I have chosen references from the work of Fukuyama (1999). Citing Christenson, she states that culture is comprised of "those commonalties around which people have developed values, norms, family life-styles, social roles and behaviors in response to historical, political, economic, and social realities" (p. 8, 9). She draws on Clinebell to define spirituality as "the human need for meaning and value in life and the desire for relationship with a transcendent power" (p. 4). Finally, she cites Worthington who states that religion is an "organized system of faith, worship, cumulative traditions, and prescribed rituals" (p. 6) carried out in a communal context. From a phenomenological standpoint, these essential elements comprise the world and life view of the individual in context. Recently, efforts have been made to distinguish spirituality from religion, as if spirituality is the recognized or universal heart of what religion is or aspires to be. Since our meaning as persons is comprised of that which we value, revere or are attached or devoted to, a strong argument can be made for a continuum of meaning that recognizes the importance of cultural, religious, and spiritual features in defining life narrative in context.

A web of meaning is woven in the context of particular cultural, spiritual and religious elements. A web of meaning is best self-defined. It could include features of age, gender, race, ethnicity, family of origin, chosen family, generational realities, spiritual and religious beliefs and practices, life style, social abilities, economic resources, sexual preference and physical and emotional gifts, limits, and characteristics. How these features comprise the strands of the web of meaning always require further elaboration. Another helpful way to grasp the nature of the web is to cite Allport's (1967) differentiation of intrinsic and extrinsic motivations of religiousness, namely from within or from outside one-self. It is artificial to separate motivations for meaning as if uncon-nected. The person by self-definition selects and is devoted to a cluster of meaning elements, often changing with context and development. For example, extrinsic identity as an American can also be heartfelt and intrinsic, a patriotic zeal that is a primary value and devotion.

LIFE NARRATIVE AS AN INTERWOVEN FABRIC

John Patton (1993) describes the present historic juncture for the pas-toral care movement as we look beyond classical (i.e., universal, deduc-tive Western) and person centered (i.e., individual, clinical pastoral) approaches. He calls for a communal contextual paradigm to incorpo-rate the resources of relational, group and societal complexity, broaden-ing the factors that are valued and studied. His call is a step towards a globalized perspective within the North American multi-spiritual/cul-tural setting and correlates with the need to investigate and incorporate spiritual and cultural dimensions of life narrative.

The anthropological perspective of ethnography is an important re-source for the study of the person in context. Grounded in the details of observation and the particular, ethnographers attend to the events and interactions that characterize a localized group, family or cluster of peo-ple over time. Patton (1993) cites Geertz that, "Understanding a people's culture exposes their normalness without reducing their particularity" (p. 15). He sees this insight as essential for shaping a pastoral understanding of the person in context. Our experience and situation as a person in context is shaped by not only how we have commonality, and thereby fit in with others, but how that fitting in has uniqueness that is no one else's, a one of a kind composite. In our particularity each of us is peculiar and odd.

To build upon this we need to see the web of meaning as comprised of universal, individual, cultural, spiritual and religious elements, de-fined by the person in transition or crisis through life narrative. No one else can recount our life narrative. Our web of meaning is comprised of a fabric of interwoven strands, our unique identity. What we value, are devoted to, and believe in is often not explicit or evident until we are in life transition or crisis when the enduring features of our life narrative, with even contrary, ambiguous or conflicted values and devotions, in the midst of chaos, come into view.

In Mayan Guatemalan villages of Tecpan, the life narrative and characteristics of the person is captured in the decorative design and fabric of the cloth out of which ceremonial clothing is made. "Traje," translated as cloth or fabric, is a weaving of threads that depict the significant elements of the traditions and locale of person, family and village, with particular emphasis upon the distinctive and creative characteristics of the wearer. The cloth is unique for each individual, even though there are common designs and colors depicting the universal and cultural features of humanity. This clothing is an imprint of the life of the person who wears it. The cloth's woven pattern and color identifies the person's uniqueness and integration into community and tradition (Hendrickson, 1995).

We might want to consider in our globalized and diverse context how the threads of identity, belief, and uniqueness comprise the cloth that is essential to our being, not to cover but to define our identity. The living human document is clothed by such a myriad identity. The story of that cloth's weaving is our life narrative. "Spiritual/cultural competency" is the capacity to read the cloth, to know one's own life narrative and hear the life narrative of another. Through the spiritual care encounter, the chaplain can bridge the gap and offer understanding and comfort in keeping with the context.

SOURCES THAT MARK THE PATH OF COMPETENCE

Multicultural counseling theorists have defined elements of competence learning by citing a five step framework, the first three initiated in the work of Pedersen (1994) and others who named and carefully defined the central value of personal awareness (1), knowledge (2), and skills (3) in multicultural competency. Personal awareness (1) is a foundational attention to one's own social identity and the impact on oneself and others, including dynamics of power. Attention to one's assumptions, values and interpersonal styles of relating deepens and enriches clinical practice and the self of the caregiver. Knowledge (2) is crucial here and is of a particular characteristic, namely information and facts about the history, experience, composition, understanding, and analysis of one's own and other's cultural identity and composition as well as the groups and forces that make up the composition.

Skills (3) are abilities to engage with oneself and others so as to acknowledge and learn about cultural dynamics in relationships and groups, especially methods of communication that facilitate growth and respect. Sevig (Fukuyama, 1999) and his colleagues developed two additional elements to the framework. Passion (4) is the dedication and caring about multicultural learning, the capacity for empathy, constructive work with feelings and the ability to risk. Action (5) is the integrating factor, the ability to relate and act in a manner consistent with awareness, knowledge, skill and passion, especially in constructive change.

Clinical pastoral education as a method of integrative learning for continuous formation in ministry practice favorably coincides with this fivefold strategy for multicultural competency development. The CPE method of action-reflection-action, also known as process education, acknowledges cognitive, emotional, and interactive dimensions integrated in the supervised clinical context. Jernigan (2000) describes the crosscultural interaction between CPE supervisor and student as a locale for mutual learning with constant translating across boundaries. Lee (2001) portrays multicultural interaction in pastoral practice as the movement of dance partners, an embodied experience calling for mutuality and an integrative learning process, the essence of CPE.

The correlation of head and heart has historically been viewed as essential to experiential learning (Note 3). The element of passion, identified in multicultural competency development, coincides with recognition of the need to join head, heart, and viscera to identify the motivation and tenaciousness required to overcome barriers and build effective communication and relationships. With passion, the chaplain can strategically speak and act for more just and equitable approaches when faced with disrespectful or demeaning action by individuals or institutions.

The pastoral care movement has until now not contributed to nor been acknowledged by the multicultural counseling field, even while an important effort to integrate spirituality with multi-cultural counseling is taking place. This is in some measure due to academic and intellectual efforts to maintain a separation of religion and the practice of ministry from the work of the behavioral sciences, lest a particular religious perspective be assumed or promoted. It also stems from the reluctance of the pastoral care movement to consider the limitations of a Judeo-Christian worldview, forged through common biblical roots and the dominance of an Euro-American perspective. Recent challenges to this tacit worldview regarding gender and racial inclusiveness are examples that mark the necessity of continuous vigilance and review. Personal and collective reluctance to address exclusionary attitudes and boundaries in a given context can be benign or malignant, in either case worthy of analysis and criticism, especially when issues of power and resource distribution weigh in.

Anthropology has long recognized the integration of religion and spirituality in cultural context, based upon observation of particular phenomena. Efforts for integrative thought address the complexity of the North American pluralistic setting and lead to practices that span disciplines. The pastoral care movement will necessarily want to strengthen, even reinvent its identity as capable of a multi-faith perspective, clarifying assumptions rooted in Judeo-Christian thought, practice, and context. The growing contention about the appropriateness of "pastoral" as the primary identity of the field, rooted in Christian biblical imagery, exemplifies the boundaries that need to be continually evaluated and re-aligned (Note 4).

FIVE STEPS FOR SPIRITUAL/ CULTURAL CHAPLAIN COMPETENCY

These conceptual sources in dialogue with experience mark a path on which I define five steps in a process of spiritual/cultural competency assessment for the chaplain. The work of others sparked this formulation. Kanuha and Ritchie (1992) developed a process for establishing diverse social work practice. Beginning with self-assessment, they emphasized the importance of relevant information and knowledge to grasp one's own cultural set and that of the client and a commitment to practice improvement and social change. These steps can be conducted by reviewing one's own practice characteristics, including limitations, and taking action to monitor and regulate oneself and to develop accountability with other practitioners.

Augsburger (1986) described characteristics to guide the pastoral counselor in developing cultural capability. He emphasized awareness of one's values and basic assumptions, a capacity to welcome and value other worldviews and contexts and a willingness to be a humane and universal citizen, open to diversity that goes beyond the known and familiar to that which is divergent and unknown. This multi-faceted awareness correlates with Pedersen (1994) and Sevig's (Fukuyama, 1999) multi-cultural characteristics of self-awareness, knowledge, skill and passion, integrated through the process of professional action. Augsburger (1986) defined interaction as "interpathy," (p. 29) a capacity whereby one temporarily takes on or enters a foreign perspective, belief and feeling state so as to see, value and believe what the other does. In order to accomplish this crucial step, the chaplain must temporarily detach from the accustomed web of reference and meaning. The utilization of imagination is necessary for this transition and entry as we shall presently see.

The Capacity to Know and Explain One's Own "Spiritual/Cultural Set," One's Own Spiritual/Cultural Groundedness

Self-awareness is the key to effective learning. As a practitioner, I am responsible to understand the spiritual and cultural characteristics of life narrative that shape my web of meaning. By grasping my values and basic assumptions, I am able to see myself in context and how I am distinguished from others both within and outside my family and community. I have derived and accumulated a distinctive spiritual/cultural set as a Euro/Anglo American male, residing and working as a privileged person in a metropolitan area, where I am part of the Protestant minority and married within a multi-religious, spiritual, and cultural blended family. The combination is as unique as my fingerprint, a web that only I can describe. The description sounds extrinsic and yet is quite intrinsic. The meaning I have woven is a particular composite of common elements that have an inside and outside attachment. As I tell my story, describing what is written in my book as a living human document, I am portraying how deep the common categories are embedded in my soul, how the fabric I wear is unique.

The Capacity to Identify Experiences and Information that Are Outside of One's Own Spiritual/Cultural References, to Identify and Learn About "Otherness"

By placing boundaries around my web of meaning, I am able within the context of a pastoral relationship to recognize the distinctive grounding of another person, the otherness of the human being before me. I need to be aware that my own assumptions blossom when I see a person of a different skin color. As a native Anglo, I might readily assume that the person is from a place far away. I need to monitor my readiness to emphasize universality, the common traits of human existence (i.e., "we are all the same or we all suffer"), that often overlooks the uniqueness that another wishes to claim. If I express common bonds too readily, I may be exercising presumption and power, interpreting as common what is distinctive or unique for someone else. To recognize the integrity of the other, postured outside my references, serves as an essential base for preparation.

The other person's story in times of transition and crisis can have an urgent and fragmented quality, as seeming disconnected pieces of a puzzle. Recognizing the broken as well as the foreign nature of the other person's context, web of meaning, is essential for me to discern what I am hearing.

The Capacity to Demonstrate Multi-Spiritual/Cultural Attitudes, Approaches, and Skills Leading to Effective Communication and Relating to Those with Other Cultural Sets

Specifically, I am called upon to engage in the monumental inner effort to temporarily set aside my own spiritual/cultural set, my web of meaning, for the purpose of crossing over boundaries into the life perspective of the other person. I may recognize that such a setting aside is not possible. I may be too anxious, confused, or preoccupied. An attitude of acceptance and respect is essential to see the other person's vantage point, through open-ended communication skills where the other person defines reality. It is a given that I have to translate not only words but also realities, requiring movement beyond my own misunderstanding and lack of reference.

I recently had the opportunity to take a deeper look on the occasion of a nurse referral to an elderly Indian Hindu woman who was eagerly waiting for her family to arrive before deciding on a routine test. She quietly indicated the importance of their participation, support, and reassurance. Taking time and energy to gain knowledge about the customs and practices of someone from another spiritual/cultural setting also calls for exploration of substantial written and human resources, as well as the time to engage this material introspectively. I will need to be informed and knowledgeable about groups and practices that I previously had no idea existed, identifying literature through library and website references to fill gaps that dramatically appear. Ka Lun Lai (2003), for example, has sensitively and forthrightly raised our awareness in ministering with Chinese patients and families.

The Capacity to Identify Contextual or Relational Barriers, as Well as One's Own Limitations, in Communication and Pastoral Practice

I attempt to face barriers and limitations, factors that are both situational and interpersonal, my discomfort zone. Not knowing the language of the other person has both literal and symbolic consequence. The nature of my own attitude, awareness, lack of skill or knowledge regarding blocks in communication skills is an important self-assessment factor. Is there someone to translate? Is communication even possible? Who is not speaking in their primary language? Effective communication is primarily my responsibility. Does my worldview allow for pluralistic reality? If I am able to identify my comfort zone and the boundaries around it, I have the possibility to identify the discomfort zone that surrounds it, an essential step in my practice learning.

The Capacity to Demonstrate Respect Within and Willingness to Learn from and Evaluate the Process of Multi-Spiritual/Cultural Interaction

Ultimately the other person is my teacher. My continuous assessment of dynamics, spiritual needs and the objectives of spiritual care are essential. Supervision and consultation with colleagues and individuals that have more experience in cross cultural care giving will enhance my learning. A context for group case consultation and/or supervision by a person with more multi-spiritual/cultural counseling experience can provide enriched competency, in mutual development and accountability and in measuring the attainment of learning. A transitional zone is possible as a learning context between my comfort and discomfort zone. A small study group of colleagues might combine articles from literature with personal and professional vignettes and prospective cases to portray personal webs of meaning and the transitional territory between comfort and discomfort zones, identifying experiences and providing feedback towards the goal of demonstrating multi-spiritual and cultural interaction and competency.

SPIRITUAL CARE CASES WHERE COMPETENCY GROWS

Case A–The patient is a 45-year-old Shiite Muslim, citizen of Yemen with a 2-year history of lymphoma. He has worked as a skilled construction worker in a large metropolitan area for over 10 years, returning to his homeland yearly. He is married to 2 women and has two families with 11 children that he supports. A recent hospitalization marks a serious advance of the disease and he has lost his hair due to chemotherapy. He has no family in the US and few visitors. Co-workers serve as his primary community and reside in a section of the city that requires 2 hours travel to the hospital.

He welcomes the chaplain to his room and describes his life crisis. He appreciates the advanced treatment he is receiving and acknowledges that such treatment would not be available to him in Yemen. In his culture and among his co-workers, brief illness is acceptable but extended illness with the diagnosis of cancer leads to loss of respect. Despite his loneliness, he acknowledges his situation as the will of Allah and has told just one friend about his illness. Daily prayers have become difficult, due to the lack of privacy.

The chaplain visiting him is a 35-year-old Korean male, married with one young child. He is active as an assistant minister in a Korean evangelical church and plans to return to his homeland upon completion of his post-graduate studies in pastoral care and counseling. His ministry as hospital chaplain provides many rich learning opportunities. He has little understanding of the Muslim faith and prayer practices, life in Yemen, and a multiple marriage situation.

A nurse makes a referral with the observation that the patient has had no visitors during an extended stay and is withdrawn. The chaplain approaches the patient to conduct a spiritual assessment and offer a relationship. Along with the initial contact, he recognizes (Step 1) that as a Korean evangelical Christian he has a well-defined context of family life within the faith community, based upon Scriptural beliefs, the working of the Spirit as well as loyalty and duty, based upon cultural tradition and respect for elders. Devotion to one wife through the sacredness of marriage is a value of central importance and a fulfillment of faith and family duty. The recognition of loneliness and personal vulnerability is socially awkward although valued in his practice.

The patient openly portrays the complexity of his web of meaning. As a devout Shiite Muslim, he has difficulty practicing his faith due to the public nature of hospitalization. As someone far from home, he experiences further alienation and misunderstanding, even though he appreciates the treatment he receives. As the husband of two wives and 11 children, he is not fulfilling his obligations as provider and cannot confide with others about his serious advanced illness and extended crisis. The chaplain (Step 2) recognizes the patient's beliefs and marital situation as formidable and challenging because of his own beliefs and understanding of marriage. He trusts his growing anxiety as an indicator of clashes that he had best explore in consultation with colleagues.

At the same time, the chaplain (Step 3) offers a relationship to the patient and takes his plight seriously. His anxiety alerts him to the need to understand beyond his current level of competency. He recognizes that he has been confronted anew by a view of God's power and role in human life that requires obedience, not questioning authority. This view challenges his view of faith maturity from a developmental perspective that he is working to utilize through his studies. Ironically, obedience to God's will correlates to a faith perspective strongly held by his own tradition. He sets objectives to reinforce the patient conducting his religious rituals, to interpret to the staff the conditions needed and to offer attention to address the loneliness and despair he sees as evident.

In doing his own inventory, the chaplain (Step 4) further acknowledges that his own view of marriage, lack of knowledge regarding the beliefs and practices of a devout Shiite Muslim and his own personal beliefs about God serve as inhibiting dynamics in the ongoing relationship. He acknowledges his lack of pastoral experience with non-Asian and non-North American patients, opening a new challenge. He sets objectives to learn from outside resources and from the patient the personal and cultural practices that he values.

The chaplain (Step 5) has identified learning value as a listener of the patient and the readiness and trust conferred by the patient in his visits. Through consultation and supervision, he develops a strategy to invite the patient to teach him more about valued traditions and beliefs. He seeks to gain clarification from the patient whether information researched regarding the Shiite Muslim faith is compatible with his experience. He inquires about the needed prayer practices and follows up with staff to facilitate privacy. The opportunity to counsel the patient is reliant upon how the patient views the complexity of his illness and it's unique meaning for his life.

Case 2–The situation centers on a 32-year-old African-Caribbean Baptist woman who is the mother of a 6-year-old boy with an advanced malignant brain tumor in the intensive care unit. She provides primary care of her son who has been sick since infancy and a 14-year-old daughter. Her husband is employed as a business manager and visits the hospital a few times a week. The course of treatment has been exhaustive. The cancer has progressed aggressively in the past few weeks and the child has lost consciousness. The mother is insistent that additional treatment be found, speaks confidently that a miracle will occur, that her constant prayer at the bedside is essential. The hospital staff is determined not to impose needless care, seeing the patient's comfort as their primary treatment goal.

The chaplain is a 45-year-old Irish American Roman Catholic sister, a native of New York, with a background as a nurse in home care and missionary work in Central America. Her spirituality has evolved during her adult life to include various forms of prayer and meditation. She finds fulfillment serving as a chaplain in a multi-cultural and spiritual hospital setting. She is troubled by the alienation that has grown between the mother and the nursing staff due to the mother's persistence and unwillingness to listen to nursing's perspective.

The chaplain visits the family continuously, hears the mother's cries of sadness and determination and openly prays with her. The chaplain discusses the mother's hope for a medical miracle, a belief based upon her early upbringing in the Caribbean where she experienced community prayer saving her younger brother from terminal disease. The pastor of her church has indicated that God is in charge, a miracle is possible, and she should not let physicians tell her otherwise. The pastor has not visited the hospital but an assistant has come weekly. The chaplain acknowledges the clash of this worldview with the scientific medical view, where lack of clinical objectivity is viewed as magical thinking, based upon psychodynamic and psychoanalytic thought.

The chaplain (Step 1) recognizes that her faith development as a professed sister and Catholic had been shaped by the various cultural settings where she has lived and ministered. She is comfortable praying with people of other faith traditions. Her worldview and experience acknowledges God's mercy through medicine and nursing and the mystery of intercession. As a Caucasian, she understands that she lives in a place of perceived and actual privilege and power.

The chaplain learns that the mother (Step 2) grew up in a rural Caribbean community that relies primarily upon God's favor and mercy, the most constant assurance in a life of poverty and uncertainty. After coming to the USA and marrying a man from her island, she joined a holiness Baptist church that believes in the power of God to overcome adversity through the Holy Spirit intervening in miraculous ways. She has had the prayer support of her church throughout the 6 years of her son's illness and through the many changes in health care services, leading to the latest oncology treatment. The pastor has reinforced a worldview that does not acknowledge and understand the value of medical science and practice. The husband is more willing to discuss options with physicians but his availability is limited.

The chaplain (Step 3) joins the patient's mother in the public expression of prayer and seeks to support her intercessions. She recognizes the intense love and attachment of the mother to the child and the increasing frustration on the part of staff who place primary value in the expertise of medical practice. Facing the death of a child touches everyone's vulnerability. The mother's web of meaning needs to be understood by others. Can the chaplain be an interpreter? With the mother's permission, the chaplain calls the pastor and leaves messages, proposing a meeting, but has no calls returned.

Based on previous experience, the chaplain (Step 4) acknowledges that she is once again confronted by the challenge of attempting to foster communication between persons in conflict with each other, whose assumptions and values are in opposition. This has been a common experience in her ministry as a missionary nurse in Central America. She recognizes that she needs to clarify with each party how they view her role, if she can serve in a conciliatory capacity or primarily support each party separately.

As the next step, the chaplain (Step 5) is able to draw from earlier life experience regarding the clash of cultural views and wants to expand her effectiveness in crisis situations. She seeks consultation and sets objectives to promote respect and patience between the parties, common language, and understanding. She broadens her circle of contacts, speaking with the attending physician and nurse team leader to convey her understanding of the emotional and spiritual reality, the web of meaning, expressed by the mother and family. The prospect of a mutually convenient conversation between all decision-makers is explored and in the process further understanding about the disparity takes place. Meanwhile, the child falls into a deeper coma and is not responsive.

DISCUSSION

The cases describe the complexity and challenge of multi-spiritual and cultural competency development, a continuous learning process essential to professional practice in a globalized and diverse health care context. The chaplain whose web of meaning is characterized with Korean and Pentecostal ties is also shaped by his experience as a married man and father. His growing understanding of human development acknowledges the complexity and integrity of the inner life and personal context. He recognizes that his relationship with the Yemeni Muslim isolated and critically ill and far from home, posits the challenge to explore his own spiritual and cultural assumptions, limitations, and barriers, his discomfort zone. Such personal reflection leads to an expansion of the comfort zone of his perspective, a transitional learning step, as he grasps the unique dilemma of the patient. His effectiveness is shaped by his capacity to grow through reflective practice.

The web of meaning for the Euro-American Catholic chaplain, with extensive background living and working in Central America, has given her experience and a reflective capacity that allows her to understand and relate to the younger African-Caribbean Baptist mother in her tragic hardship, keeping vigil by her comatose son. The mother's desperate insistence on a miracle is borne of the spiritual/cultural web in which meaning shapes reality. The chaplain seeks to bridge the conflict and impasse with hospital staff by moving back and forth between participants and fostering recognition of the disparities. Her contribution focuses upon contextual barriers emerging from assumptions and attitudes that will not necessarily be overcome but will be useful through retrospective consultation in the clinical setting. In such a stand off, a breakthrough is possible as staff search their attitudes and actively learn about the web of meaning held by the mother and how it is connected to her family and their faith community.

In this article, groundwork has been identified that can serve as the basis for continuous professional learning by spiritual care providers in health care settings to develop spiritual/cultural competency. Chaplains in hospitals can utilize process learning through clinical pastoral education methodology whereby an open ended framework for spiritual care practice seeks to meet the surprising and unexpected challenges brought about by the globalized diversity in our communities. An understanding of the person as a vital and living human document, clothed in a distinctively woven fabric, a composite of meaning based on personal and collective history, is also absolutely basic. The contrast and complexity within a person makes each of us a unique composite of characteristics shaped by our life narrative and heritage.

Competency relies upon recognition that the existing spiritual/cultural limitations of the Judeo-Christian perspective embedded in our society, significantly influences and confines our approach. We need to grasp the web of meaning that characterizes individual reality in responding to the web of meaning embodied in the person we serve. In facing the pluralistic nature of spiritual care giving, we are called to address and set aside subtle as well as overt attempts at conversion, to influence the person to think or believe as we do.

CONCLUSION

Spiritual/cultural competency integrates elements of self-awareness, understanding and interactive skill that acknowledges caring and commitment to relationships in which learning leads the way. In outlining spiritual/cultural competency, five steps or dimensions have been explored. I need, first of all, to grasp my own spiritual/cultural set, the web of meaning that shapes my reality. What characterizes my view of myself in the world, my beliefs and devotions? Am I, secondly, able and committed to exploring realities outside my own, to acknowledge the countless diversity of "otherness" or do I primarily seek reinforcement of what I know? Thirdly, am I capable of attitudes and approaches that foster interaction and relationships with others so that their distinctiveness as a carrier of meaning is evident? Fourthly, in such an interaction, am I able to identify the limits and barriers that emerge in my spiritual care giving? Do I see the discomfort zones and have ways to facilitate transitions to communication? And, lastly, do I have settings and methods for ongoing learning, to find consultation and expertise so as to continuously deepen my capacity in search of spiritual/cultural competency? I have more to plumb from my personal narrative and the rich field of interaction with those I serve. My search as a spiritual care provider for spiritual/cultural competency is one that is open ended, shaped and revised by the person to person encounter with the stranger and the web of meaning the stranger has woven. The depth I find and the mystery I sense reminds me that this endeavor is inherently sacred.

AUTHOR NOTE

Robert Anderson is an ACPE chaplain supervisor and staff chaplain who has served in four metropolitan hospital settings over the past 32 years. Ministry in three small cities, each community with a rich multi-spiritual and cultural composition, has now given way to the living laboratory of New York City, his hometown. Through relationships with patients, their families and loved ones and with medical and hospital staff, he has come to recognize the necessity and exhilaration of learning and growing with spiritual and cultural diversity. Through increasing ties with religious communities in the various cities (one with eight ethnically different Eastern Orthodox denominations), he grew in his attentiveness to cultural and religious approaches, values and practices for people in crisis.

Anderson grew up in an Euro-American nuclear family residing in city neighborhoods where he was in a minority of 10 percent. A local Reformed Protestant congregation became an extended family, a cosmopolitan church where distinct heritages and diversity, albeit Caucasian, were openly acknowledged and celebrated. Marriage in a blended family has brought further enrichment. The return to New York City led to a more careful and open study of spiritual and cultural competency resources.

NOTES

1. Dr. Sam Beck, valued mentor, colleague, and social and cultural anthropologist at the College of Human Ecology, Cornell University, first introduced me to this valuable phrase.

2. Anton Boisen (1953) cited the phrase in this article, used frequently in his teaching and lecturing. Also see Gerkin (1984), p. 200, footnote 1 for more on the phrase's origin.

3. Charles Hall (1992) utilized the tension between head and heart, ideas and emotions, to recount the history of the clinical pastoral education movement. Acknowledging the viscera (gut or bowels) as a third tension to me gives passion, the seat of power and death, its place as a force in process learning.

4. Larry Austin's (1999) editorial in The Journal Of Pastoral Care aptly describes the query as to whether "pastoral" is inclusive enough to describe the proliferating and complex field of spirituality, spiritual care practice, and research. No alternative has yet appeared to name and bless the field.

REFERENCES

Allport, Gordon. (1967). Behavioral science, religion, and mental health. In D. Belgum (Ed.), *Religion and medicine: Essays on meaning, values, and health* (pp. 83-95). Ames IA: Iowa State University Press.

Augsburger, David W. (1986). *Pastoral counseling across cultures.* Philadelphia: The Westminster Press.

Austin, Larry J. (1999). "Guest editorial-Spirituality rediscovered, " *The Journal of Pastoral Care,* 53,1, 3-5.

Boisen, Anton. (1953). "Clinical training in theological education: The period of beginnings," *Chicago Theological Seminary Register.*

Fukuyama, Mary. (1999). *Integrating Spirituality into Multicultural Counseling.* Thousand Oaks: Sage Publications.

Geertz, Clifford. (1973). *The Interpretation of Cultures.* New York: Basic Books.

Gerkin, Charles. (1984). *The living human document.* Nashville: Abingdon Press.

Hall, Charles E. (1992). *Head and Heart.* Journal of Pastoral Care Publications.

Hendrickson, Carol. (1995). *Weaving identities, construction of dress and self in a highland Guatemala town.* Austin: University of Texas Press.

Jernigan, Homer L. (2000). "Clinical pastoral education with students from other cultures: The role of the supervisor." *Journal of Pastoral Care,* 54(2); 135-146.

Ka Lun Lai, Alan. (2003). "Dragon talk: Providing pastoral care for chinese immigrants." *Journal of Pastoral Care,* 57, 45-52.

Kanuha, Valli, & Richie, Beth. (1992). "Six steps to creating and maintaining culturally diverse social work practice." Unpublished manuscript.

Kluckhohn, Clyde, & Murray, Henry. (1948). *Personality in nature, society, and culture.* New York: Alfred A Knopf.

Lee, K. Samuel. (2001). "Becoming multicultural dancers: The pastoral practitioner in a multicultural society." *Journal of Pastoral Care,* 55, 389-396.

Patton, John. (1993). *Pastoral care in context.* Louisville: Westminster/John Knox Press.

Pedersen, Paul. (1994). *A handbook for developing multicultural awareness.* Alexandria: American Counseling Assoc.

Sue, Derald Wing et al. (1998). *Multicultural counseling competencies.* Thousand Oaks, Calif.: Sage Publications.

Thornton, Edward. (1970). *Professional education for ministry: A history of clinical pastoral education.* Nashville: Abingdon Press.

Cultural Diversity in Pastoral Care

Mary A. Fukuyama, PhD
Todd D. Sevig, PhD

SUMMARY. Fukuyama and Sevig are counseling psychologists who have a particular interest in the integration of spirituality into multicultural counseling and training. In this article the authors address the complexity of integrating religious and cultural diversity and spirituality into chaplaincy care in the context of an increasingly diverse society. By posing a series of questions, the authors systematically clarify definitions and meanings of culture, spirituality, cultural diversity and multiculturalism, multicultural and spiritual competencies in counseling, and ethical considerations. The authors discuss clinical applications in the context of a "spirituality and health movement," and provide suggestions for continuing professional development. The authors support the notion that multicultural engagement is spiritually synergistic, and en-

---

Mary A. Fukuyama is Clinical Professor and Licensed Psychologist, Counseling Center, University of Florida, Gainesville, FL (E-mail: fukuyama@counsel.ufl.edu).

Todd D. Sevig is Director, Counseling and Psychological Services, University of Michigan, Ann Arbor, MI (E-mail: tdsevig@umich.edu).

[Haworth co-indexing entry note]: "Cultural Diversity in Pastoral Care." Fukuyama, Mary A., and Todd D. Sevig. Co-published simultaneously in *Journal of Health Care Chaplaincy* (The Haworth Pastoral Press, an imprint of The Haworth Press, Inc.) Vol. 13, No. 2, 2004, pp. 25-42; and: *Ministry in the Spiritual and Cultural Diversity of Health Care: Increasing the Competency of Chaplains* (ed: Robert G. Anderson, and Mary A. Fukuyama) The Haworth Pastoral Press, an imprint of The Haworth Press, Inc., 2004, pp. 25-42. Single or multiple copies of this article are available for a fee from The Haworth Document Delivery Service [1-800-HAWORTH, 9:00 a.m. - 5:00 p.m. (EST). E-mail address: docdelivery@haworthpress.com].

Digital Object Identifier: 10.1300/J080v13n02_02

courage health care providers to communicate across professional disciplines to broaden and enrich discourse on these topics.

KEYWORDS. Multiculturalism, multicultural and spiritual counseling comptencies

INTRODUCTION

"Truly, it is in the darkness that one finds the light, so when we are in sorrow, then this light is nearest of all to us." Meister Eckhart (cited in Cameron, 2002, p. 171)

The work of healthcare chaplains is a sacred calling. To be genuinely present with patients during times of health crises and possibly facing death is spiritual work. Hospital settings typically do not emphasize spirituality because the biomedical model of healthcare strives to be efficient and objective. The role of the chaplain is complex, negotiating multiple realities of physicians, nursing staff, families, and various religious and culturally diverse traditions. Yet, it is precisely at this juncture that the chaplain is in a position to hold a space for the "light" referred to by Meister Eckart. While there may be agreement on the importance of light (hope, spirit, God, love, transcendence) in times of darkness, how the light is perceived, experienced, and named varies by diverse cultural and religious traditions. The question of how cultural diversity impacts the work of the healthcare chaplain is the focus of this article.

As we begin our discussion, we highlight the following points:

- The United States is a religiously diverse nation, with perhaps over 2,000 identifiable expressions of religion and spiritual paths (Creedon, 1998).
- Spiritual and religious beliefs and practices are common to humanity and are intimately related to health, sickness, death, and healing in most cultures. Whereas it is not possible for counselors

or clergy to be experts on all religions or spiritual beliefs, it is important that they have a basic understanding of cultural and religious diversity (Fukuyama & Sevig, 1999).
- Spiritual and religious beliefs are imbedded in culture, and may be discussed in the context of understanding the "worldviews" of culturally diverse clients or patients (Sue and Sue, 2003).
- Consideration of diverse spiritual and religious beliefs and practices may serve as a catalyst for the caregiver's personal growth and clarification of values (Fukuyama & Sevig, 1999).

We (co-authors) have organized this article to address a series of questions: (1) What is meant by cultural diversity? (2) What is meant by spiritual or religious diversity? (3) How is learning about cultural diversity relevant to spirituality? (4) What does it mean to be multiculturally and spiritually competent? (5) What are some clinical examples of cultural diversity in the context of pastoral care? (6) What are some ethical considerations in working with culturally diverse populations? (7) How can chaplains develop further their skills in multicultural competency?

(1) What is meant by cultural diversity? We have adapted an inclusive definition of culture. Culture consists ". . . of commonalties around which people have developed values, norms, family life-styles, social roles, and behaviors in response to historical, political, economic, and social realities" (Christensen, 1989, p. 275). Everyone has culture and cultural identities include communication styles, language, and socio-demographic features such as race, ethnicity, language, religion, social class, physical abilities, sexual orientation, age, nationality, and more. It is easier to be aware of one's own culture through contrast with another's culture. For example, while traveling in Latin America, I (Fukuyama) became more aware of a Euro-American Protestant work ethic in my family upbringing (i.e., to be "doing" vs. "being"), in contrast with a more relaxed socializing style that was more present-centered.

It has been important in our experience in multicultural training to address two primary dynamics: one is to explore the similarities and differences between cultures (values, customs, and worldview), and the second is to understand the concepts of power and privilege (e.g., systemic access to resources). As proponents of multiculturalism, we acknowledge that we live in a world that has more than one point of view about what constitutes "reality." Multiculturalism means that many cultures, many worldviews, many languages, many values, and many customs, exist and serve to form human communities. Secondly, it means seeking common ground, respecting differences, and working for social justice in a system that historically has kept various groups from access to resources and power through the "-isms," e.g., sexism, racism, heterosexism, and other forms of oppression. Thus, questioning and analyzing power is an underlying theme in multicultural work. In the remainder of this article, we use the terms cultural diversity and multiculturalism interchangeably.

We make a distinction between cultural values and morality. Cultural values typically refer to social constructs that vary along a continuum, such as "individualistic vs. collectivistic" cultures. For example, in the United States, we tend to value the individual over the group. Most Latin American cultures value the group (family) over the individual. In this case, we have cultural differences; neither is inherently right or wrong. Thus, the concept of cultural relativism, "it depends upon the cultural context." This line of thinking is different from moral values, which inherently implies a right-wrong distinction. Religion by definition includes codes of ethics and rules that govern behavior (Swindler & Mojzes, 2000). Sometimes religious values are used to reinforce cultural norms, such as viewing "the man as head of the household" as sacrosanct. Sometimes religious leaders are critical of cultural relativism because it does not uphold a particular morality (right-wrong). Dealing with value differences (both cultural and moral) can sometimes present ethical dilemmas. We will discuss this further in the section on ethical considerations.

(2) What is meant by spiritual or religious diversity? It is difficult to reach a consensus on what is meant by spirituality, but we offer some working definitions. In the counseling profession, we have adapted the following definition of spirituality from the Association for Spiritual, Ethical, and Religious Values in Counseling (ASERVIC), a member association of the American Counseling Association.

Spirituality is "the animating force in life, represented by such images as breath, wind, vigor, and courage. Spirituality is the infusion and drawing out of spirit in one's life. It is an innate capacity and tendency to move towards knowledge, love, meaning, hope, transcendence, connectedness, and compassion. It includes one's capacity for creativity, growth, and the development of a values system. Spirituality encompasses the religious, spiritual, and transpersonal." ("Summit results," 1995)

From the pastoral counseling tradition, Clinebell (1995) defines spirituality as the human need for meaning and value in life and the desire for relationship with a transcendent power. He further defines spiritual growth as that which "aims at the enhancement of our realistic hope, our meanings, our values, our inner freedom, our faith systems, our peak experiences, and our relationship with God" (p. 19).

How is spirituality different from religion? We distinguish spirituality as it relates to a personal experience of the Sacred. Religion may be defined as an organized system of faith, worship, cumulative traditions, and prescribed rituals (Worthington, 1989). However, we honor that all world religions are inspired by Spirit and that individuals often need to share their personal spirituality with others. From a cultural standpoint, we see spirituality as the essence and religion as being the cultural container which shapes group identity and customs (Artress, 1995).

Religious or spiritual diversity refers to the many different expressions of faith, beliefs, practices, and meanings given to spirituality, religion, and the transpersonal (literally meaning "beyond the person"). Religious pluralism has increased in the United States of America through immigration patterns over the past century (Hoge, 1996). Changing immigration patterns include increased numbers of Muslims, Latino Catholics, and Southeast Asians, for example, see *http://www. pluralism.org/about/mission.php)*. Additionally, diversity between and within religious organizations (e.g., mainstream denominations) can be observed by contrasting conservative and liberal values and including ethnic variations (e.g., African Methodist Episcopal, Korean Baptist). The World Wide Web provides information on religious and ecumenical movements that are useful for personal learning as well as in the classroom (see *http://www.awesome library.org/Classroom/Social_ Studies/Multicultural/Religious_Diversity.html.* and also *http://www. religioustolerance.org/* and *http://religiousmovements.lib.virginia.edu/)*. The interweaving of cultural and religious diversity may be a hallmark of "New American" spirituality, according to Elizabeth Lesser (1999), co-founder of the Omega Institute, a holistic education retreat center. More and more Americans now adapt their individual spiritual paths from the world's religious traditions.

Although we are a culturally and religiously diverse nation, the "dominant paradigm" continues to be Judeo-Christian, with the emphasis upon Christian. For example, national holidays tend to include Christmas and the weekly "day of rest" tends to be Sunday (whereas Fridays and Saturdays are days of worship in Islam and Judaism respectively). Religious affiliation is an important component of cultural identity. The challenge for caregivers is to be comfortable in their own cultural and religious identity and open to working with and understanding different cultural and religious worldviews (Frame, 2003; Miller, 2002).

(3) How is learning about cultural diversity relevant to spirituality? We have proposed that a synergy takes place when one experiences cultural diversity. Consider a metaphor of a window that has reflective qualities to it. Looking through the window of diversity, one sees difference; new ways of doing things or of being in the world; one's worldview becomes expanded. This seems to meet a natural human impulse, to transcend oneself and one's situation

(hence great interest in travel and sojourning). At the same time, cultural diversity provides a mirror in which one sees self (beliefs and customs). Through this self-reflective process a greater sense of self can emerge, a clearer understanding of one's beliefs, for example. We see this interaction effect as being like a spiral, an expansion of consciousness, connections with others and connections with self and community. Many persons who engage in this consciousness-raising process also become aware of social justice issues and incorporate social action into their learning process.

Engaging in multicultural training is enhanced by attention to spiritual values. We have found that incorporating spiritual and multicultural values enriches the window-mirror exercise mentioned above. Both have the potential to contribute toward an expansion of one's worldview and deepening of faith. Knowledge of differing world views has a two-fold effect: "I have a clearer idea of who I am now, because I know who I am NOT." And secondly, even though we are different, we are also similar, e.g., we worship God, even though God is called different names. In realizing these connections, a feeling of separateness is gradually lessened. A paradoxical effect of clarifying and softening cultural boundaries happens simultaneously.

Experience has shown that people struggle with the dilemmas of understanding the meaning of diversity and multiculturalism. Cultural conflicts are stressful and a multicultural society is more likely to be dynamic, challenging, and changing. This is true for the United States as a nation, and also for the world community as globalization becomes a reality (see *http://www.unesco.org/most/rr1.htm*). Clearly, unlearning racism, confronting internalized oppression, truly valuing difference, and taking risks to build alliances are formidable and painful tasks. Fortunately, spiritual qualities can assist the process of multiculturalism (see Table 1). The interaction of faith, creativity, patience, humor, flexibility, and the ability to detach or let go of one's point of view (even momentarily) will assist the process of becoming multiculturally skilled. Feelings of love and compassion for humanity ("we are all connected") increase the chances of working through difficult cultural differences. A

TABLE 1. Comparison of Spiritual and Multicultural Values

Spiritual Values	Multicultural Values
Connectedness w/others	Cultural similarities
Compassion & love	Cultural differences
Relationship outside of self	Movement from ethnocentrism towards cultural pluralism
Social Justice	Dealing with issues of oppression, advocacy
Faith	Flexibility & patience
Grace, intimacy, creativity	Commitment & humor
Sacredness & mystery	Tolerance for ambiguity
Detachment	Observational skills
Paradox	Bicultural & multicultural skills

Fukuyama, M. & Sevig, T. *Integrating Spirituality into Multicultural Counseling*, p. 75, Copyright © 1999 by Sage Publications, Inc. Reprinted with Permission of Sage Publications, Inc.

reciprocal cycle of learning can yield benefits to both the multicultural and spiritual seeker. Thus, we suggest that multicultural learning fosters spiritual evolvement, and that spiritual evolvement strengthens the multicultural learning process.

(4) *What does it mean to be multiculturally and spiritually competent?* The counseling profession has developed guidelines for spiritual and multicultural competencies. Recent ASERVIC guidelines for spiritual competencies ask counselors, in part, to be able to "describe religious and spiritual beliefs and practices in a cultural context . . . engage in self-exploration . . . demonstrate sensitivity to and acceptance of a variety of religious and/or spiritual expressions in the client's communication . . . and identify the limits of one's understanding of a client's spiritual expression." (Full list of competencies are available at *http://www.counseling.org/aservic/ Spirituality_Competencies.html*)

These competencies are similar to multicultural counseling competencies which ask counselors to be self-aware, knowledgeable about different cultural traditions, able to understand the client's worldview, and skilled in communicating with and helping diverse clients. We rec-

TABLE 2. Framework for Multicultural Competency

PERSONAL AWARENESS   *(Definition: awareness of self as a member of social groups and of self in a system of oppression)*

- aware of the impact of my social identity group memberships on myself
- able to verbalize and act on my awareness of how my social identity group memberships impact others
- aware of the impact of my interpersonal style on others
- aware of and able to articulate my values
- able to recognize areas in which I need to grow

KNOWLEDGE   *(Definition: information/knowledge)*

- knowledge of multiple groups histories and experiences in this country
- recognize the history of oppression
- recognize the importance of histories of various social groups
- models, conceptual frameworks, and terminology

SKILLS   *(Definition: facilitating change in individuals, groups, and systems; managing critical incidents; strategic analysis/action)*

- provide feedback in a direct manner; receive feedback in an open manner
- recognize group dynamics in a manner that includes multicultural factors
- address oppressive behavior in a manner that allows others to hear and which is based on behavioral data
- able to intervene in group situations and ask probing/educational questions

PASSION
(Definition: deep personal reason for caring about/doing this work and the ability to articulate this to others)

- ability to communicate compassion and empathy
- ability to communicate/share strong feelings of anger, fear, love, excitement, guilt, sorrow, etc. when appropriate
- ability to lead with heart (in addition to head)

ACTION *(Definition: ability to behave/act in a manner consistent with awareness, knowledge, skills, passion)*

- can interrupt oppression
- can take proactive measures against oppression
- can identify opportunities for action

ommend the guidelines for multicultural competency that are presented in Table 2.

Hoopes (1979) describes a multicultural learning process for a pluralistic world. The stages of consciousness-raising begin at ethnocentrism ("my way is the right way") and evolve through a sensitization process of awareness, understanding, acceptance, appreciation, and selective adoption of cultural skills (assimilation, adaptation, biculturalism, multiculturalism). Consciousness-raising also involves a deepening and expanding spiral of self development. Another such model is the "optimal theory applied to identity development" OTAID model (described in Fukuyama & Sevig, 1999) in which one progresses through various phases of identity development, concurrently expanding one's views of self and others in an inclusive way. The latter phase involves spiritual connection with all living beings.

Engaging in multicultural learning related to religion and healthcare may test some fundamental notions of 'truth' or 'my way is the right way,' or 'the way I was raised is *the* way.' Part of this exploration is to understand the cultural influences that have affected how one understands religion. For example, it is helpful to know the difference between basic Islamic religious tenets, and how the various cultural factors in any particular Muslim country have affected the practice of these tenets throughout history. This seems particularly timely in today's world in which religious beliefs are intertwined with politics, history, and international relations.

One of the tensions involved in providing multiculturally sensitive delivery of service is to know "when to travel" or "leave home," (i.e., one's comfort zone). The goal is to be strong in one's own evolving sense of identity (more specifically, one's identity make-up or profile) and yet being able to work with, and to take the perspective of the 'other' in providing service. There are a number of steps involved in this: (a) having a deep understanding of one's own personal biases/stereotypes/preconceptions before working with another person; (b) having a general sense/understanding of the cultural influences that may be affecting the person you are working with; (c) engaging in some sense of assessment of how cultural factors may be influencing the person you are working with; (d) knowing your own cultural influences and how they have impacted your practice as a chaplain (or any of the helping professions), and (e) being able to attach language and behaviors that are consistent with points a-d.

(5) *What are some clinical examples of cultural diversity in the context of pastoral care?* Cultural diversity also includes the worldviews that are prevalent in biomedicine. In a recent conference on integrating spirituality in healthcare, Dr. Christina Puchalski (2003) noted that physicians' worldviews toward medicine influence how they view the patients with whom they are working. She posited three possible attitudes: Medicine as "helping," which views "life as weak"; medicine as "fixing a problem," which views "life as broken"; and finally, medicine as "serving," which views "life as a whole." These same underlying worldviews or fundamental assumptions on life can be applied to pastoral care, that is, how do chaplains define their roles in relation to the patient, and how does that fit into the larger healthcare system?

In terms of understanding cultural diversity, healthcare providers and chaplains need to be aware of their own worldviews as well as understanding the patients' perspectives. Traditional Western medicine takes an allopathic approach to treating disease; literally it means "treating sickness oppositely." That is, the treatment counteracts symptoms with medicine that creates an "opposite" to the symptom (e.g., treating asthma with medicine that dilates the bronchial tubes). The strengths of Western medicine are in the area of antibiotics, treating emergencies, and surgical interventions. However, the trend towards specializations in biomedicine promotes high levels of technical skills but lack of awareness of the "whole person" and of the interrelatedness of mind-body-spirit. Sometimes the chaplain may be called to treat the "whole person" while the biomedical system is focused on fixing "problems." For example, the decision to do an organ transplant to extend life may make technical sense, but not emotional or moral sense for someone who is preparing for death.

How does spirituality interact with health, illness, and healing? These questions are just beginning to be explored in a newly formed "spirituality and health movement in healthcare" (see *http://www. spiritualityandhealth.ufl.edu/;* Koenig, 1997; Levin, 2001). Spiritual dimensions related to illness, health and healing, such as the healing power of prayer, beliefs around dying and death, are topics naturally suited for the chaplain's attention. In some cases, spiritual beliefs and practices may be foreign to the caregiver, such as in the case history of a Hmong child treated for epilepsy in a California hospital (Fadiman, 1997). Both religious and folk beliefs often contribute to explanations of illnesses in traditional Latino and Asian families (see Fukuyama & Sevig, 2002). The cultural complexities in our country increase exponentially when considering new arrivals (immigrants, refugees) in addition to other diversity factors (religion, sexual orientation, socioeconomic class, to name a few).

One way to address the complexities of the whole person in a cultural context is to elicit the patient's story. For example, one innovation is found in the "narrative medicine" program, started by Dr. Rita Charon (2002) at Columbia University. This program trains physicians to elicit the patient's story about their illness. There is something basically healing and honoring of the person when someone takes time to listen deeply.

Similarly, medical anthropologist Arthur Kleinman has developed sample questions of inquiry in what he calls an "explanatory model" for illness:

1. What do you call the problem?
2. What do you think has caused the problem?
3. Why do you think it started when it did?
4. What do you think the sickness does? How does it work?
5. How severe is the sickness? Will it have a short or long course?
6. What kind of treatment do you think the patient should receive? What are the most important results you hope she [the patient] receives from this treatment?
7. What are the chief problems the sickness has caused?

8. What do you fear most about the sickness? (cited in Fadiman, 1997, pp. 260-261)

Chaplains may adapt some of these questions with their patients when exploring the meaning of illness with them.

Other clinical situations that beckon for multicultural awareness include situations of differing religious beliefs related to death, dying, and customs for handling the body after death, ethical decision-making related to medical interventions, understanding the cultural meaning and management of pain, and integrating multiple modalities for healing.

(6) What are some ethical considerations in working with culturally diverse populations? One will likely encounter ethical concerns and tensions when immersed in a culturally diverse setting (Pack-Brown & Williams, 2003). One point of tension along this journey is working with the notion that being multiculturally competent does not have to imply that one is being 'weak' in one's own beliefs and values. For example, one can have strong Christian beliefs, values, and cultural identifiers and competently work with someone who is Jewish, Islamic, or from another faith or religious tradition. To be effective, however, requires following several key points: (a) not proselytizing from one's own perspective; (b) being aware of power and privilege issues in how religion has been enacted in this country (e.g., Protestant Christian traditions being seen as the norm); (c) having a pluralistic worldview-no one tradition has the 'corner on the truth,' and (d) avoiding an "either/or" dichotomy in viewing these issues, and embracing a "both/and" perspective, e.g., "I can be a strong Christian, *and value someone else's experience in being Islamic."*

It is important to recognize value conflicts that may involve an ethical dilemma for the caregiver. Among the more obvious issues, such as abortion, caregivers need to be able to delineate boundaries that are consistent with their personal values as well as providing for respectful patient care. Dealing with issues of sexuality and sexual orientation may challenge religious principles for some. The primary ethical concern, however, is "to do no harm" to the client or patient, and if the caregiver's biases prevent good care, it is best to refer.

Aside from the obvious cases, however, caregivers can be oblivious to their biases. For example, what is your position on "acculturation" or "assimilation" into mainstream culture? Should the patient be expected to give up his or her folk beliefs for modern medicine? What if a patient insists on keeping string bracelets on her wrists or a medicine pouch around his neck for spiritual protection? What if the doctor insists on a patient making a medical decision and the family insists that the husband of the patient makes the decision? Such cultural nuances often require consultation with a medical team that can discern a culturally sensitive response. Generally speaking, it is desirable if one can accommodate the "both/and" of cultural complexity instead of forcing a dichotomous choice (either/or). It may be more helpful to incorporate *both* traditional *and* alternative modes of healing, for example, or at least some cultural compromise.

(7) *How can chaplains develop further their skills in multicultural competency?* What is involved in training and learning multicultural competency? Ironically, most senior level practitioners lack training in this area. Graduate programs are just now integrating cultural diversity training. Our experience has been that acquiring multicultural skills is a lifelong learning process. Here are some basic ways to begin and to continue the process: attend Continuing Education programs, participate in supervision and training groups, engage in peer supervision and case discussion, conduct community visits, interview cultural informants, participate in consciousness raising discussions, and do personal racial identity work (see Adams, Bell, & Griffin, 1997). Other ideas include attending cultural events, experiencing "being the other" in both minority and majority roles, and reading books and viewing videos

with multicultural themes (for learning exercises see Pack-Brown & Williams, 2003).

In an article describing a multicultural training seminar for graduate students, Sevig and Etzkorn (2001) outline three aspects they consider essential to a multicultural learning process. First, recognition of the complexity of multiple identities is necessary; a white woman's experience is different than a white man's experience of multiculturalism-by only focusing on 'white' misses the complexity of the full experiences. Second, power dynamics need to be addressed directly versus being 'under the surface.' It is helpful when privilege is examined in personal, cultural, and institutional ways, and ways of talking about this are identified. Third, a journey is solid when it incorporates both universal and culture-specific approaches-again, this does not need to be an 'either/or' enterprise.

CONCLUSION

This article addresses the complexity of integrating religious and cultural diversity, spirituality, and health into chaplaincy care. Although we whole-heartedly endorse multicultural work, we also offer a few words of caution. When considering cultural diversity, our experience has taught us that the ideal is to be self-motivated and an active learner, and at the same time, to be aware of balancing the need for "challenge and support." Learning too much too quickly about diversity can be overwhelming, stressful, and/or cause one to be defensive or scattered. Too much focus on difference may contribute to feelings of disconnection and loss of contact with one's own traditions. A more natural life long progression, however, leads to work that can be stimulating, exciting, and energizing as one lets go of stereotypes, acquires new knowledge, and breaks down social barriers.

Our way of tempering this process is to follow the maxim that describes an intention of spirituality and religion, "to comfort the distressed and distress the comfortable" (Scherer, 1961, p. 44). We recognize and honor that doing multicultural work requires effort and commitment, patience and humor, curiosity and risk-taking. We encourage challenge and support! Just as the faith journey is rewarding through years of deepening experiences, the multicultural journey is rewarding, expansive, and enriching.

AUTHOR NOTE

Todd Sevig and Mary Fukuyama are counseling practitioners in university counseling centers and have published work in the area of integrating spirituality into multicultural counseling (Fukuyama & Sevig, 1999). Both share a commitment to infusing multiculturalism in their work and see this as a lifelong process. Just as faith development has been described as a journey, the development of multicultural counseling competency is a journey that can be described as having highs and lows, progress and slippage, epiphanies, and uncertainties. This article is another step in the journey, one of exploring the intricacies of spiritual, religious, and cultural diversity in the context of chaplaincy healthcare.

Both Todd and Mary have background experience with clergy, in that their fathers were Protestant ministers and chaplains who served in the prison system and VA respectively. Todd summarized his interests in these words, "I have been struck by how naturally cultural diversity, religion, and health fit together and yet how simultaneously they seem 'worlds apart.' I will probably spend the majority of my life attempting to reconcile this irony. My father was a Protestant minister and a chaplain for a men's prison. I watched him as he moved in and out of various settings (the church, the prison, hospitals, and home visits). As I got older and moved in the direction of psychology, I tended to separate or compartmentalize religion, psychology, and healthcare. However, at this point, I seek dialogue, collaboration, and integration, by having these disciplines learn from each other. My hope is that this article represents one small strand to this end."

Mary summarized her interests with the following observation. "I see poignant similarities between the role of pastoral counselor and psychologist . . . a desire to help, a search for meaning and purpose, a concern for privacy of the personal, and a connection to community tempered by role status, that is, belonging yet slightly set apart. I never thought I would follow my father's footsteps professionally, but I certainly share in the above qualities of life in my role as a university counseling psychologist. Given that I grew up as a child of a "preacher," I am comfortable with religious discourse, and welcome every opportunity to intermingle psychological insights with religious and spiritual awareness. My hope is that our commitment to infusing multiculturalism in counseling will benefit the readers of this article on integrating cultural diversity in pastoral care."

REFERENCES

Adams, M., Bell, L.A., & Griffin, P. (Eds.). (1997). *Teaching for diversity and social justice: A sourcebook.* New York: Routledge.

Artress, L. (1995). Walking a sacred path: *Rediscovering the labyrinth as a spiritual tool.* New York: Riverhead Books.

Cameron, J. (2002). *The artist's way: A spiritual path to higher creativity.* New York: Jeremy P. Tarcher/Putnam.

Charon, R. (2002). *Stories matter: The role of narrative in medical ethics.* New York: Routledge.

Christensen, C. P. (1989). Cross-cultural awareness development: A conceptual model. *Counselor Education and Supervision, 28,* 270-289.

Clinebell, H. (1995). *Counseling for spiritually empowered wholeness: A hope-centered approach.* New York: The Haworth Pastoral Press.

Creedon, J. (1998, July-August). God with a million faces. *Utne Reader,* 42-48.

Fadiman, A. (1997). *The spirit catches you and you fall down: A Hmong child, her American doctors, and the collision of two cultures.* New York: Farrar, Straus, & Giroux.

Frame, M.W. (2003). *Integrating religion and spirituality into counseling: A comprehensive approach.* Pacific Grove, CA: Brooks/Cole.

Fukuyama, M.A., & Sevig, T.D. (1999). *Integrating spirituality into multicultural counseling.* Thousand Oaks, CA: Sage Publications.

Fukuyama, M.A., & Sevig, T.D. (2002). Spirituality in counseling across cultures: Many rivers to the sea. In P. B. Pedersen, J. G. Draguns, W. J. Lonner, & J. E. Trimble (Eds). *Counseling across cultures* (5th ed.) (pp. 273-295). Thousand Oaks, CA: Sage.

Hoge, D. (1996). Religion in America: The demographics of belief and affiliation. In E. P. Shafranske (Ed.), *Religion and the clinical practice of psychology* (pp. 21-41). Washington, DC: American Psychological Association.

Hoopes, D.S. (1979). Intercultural communication concepts and the psychology of intercultural experience. In M.D. Pusch (Ed.), *Multicultural education: A cross-cultural training approach.* LaGrange Park, IL: Intercultural Network, Inc.

Koenig, H.G. (1997). *Is religion good for your health? The effects of religion on physical and mental health.* Binghamton, NY: The Haworth Press, Inc.

Lesser, E. (1999) *The seeker's guide: Making your life a spiritual adventure.* New York: Villard.

Levin, J. (2001). *God, faith, and health: Exploring the spirituality-healing connection.* New York: John Wiley.

Miller, G. (2002). *Incorporating spirituality in counseling and psychotherapy: Theory and technique.* New York: John Wiley & Sons.

Pack-Brown, S.P., & Williams, C.B. (2003). *Ethics in a multicultural context.* Thousand Oaks, CA: Sage.

Pulchaski, C. (2003, March 27-28). Spirituality and healing in medicine: A multicultural approach. Spirituality and Health Conference, Indianapolis.

Scherer, P. (1961). *Love is a spendthrift.* New York: Harper.Sevig, T., & Etzkorn, J. (2001), Transformative training: A year-long multicultural counseling seminar for graduate students. *Journal of Multicultural Counseling & Development, 29*(1), 57-72.

Swindler, L.J., & Mojzes, P. (2000). *The study of religion in an age of global dialogue.* Philadelphia: Temple University Press. Summit results in formation of spirituality competencies. (December, 1995). *Counseling Today* (p. 30).

Worthington, E. L. (1989). Religious faith across the life span: Implications for counseling and research. *The Counseling Psychologist, 17*, 555-612.

RESPONSES TO:
ANDERSON, FUKUYAMA, AND SEVIG

Toward Multicultural Competencies for Pastoral/Spiritual Care Providers in Clinical Settings: Response to Anderson, Fukuyama, and Sevig

K. Samuel Lee, PhD

K. Samuel Lee, PhD, is Visiting Professor of Pastoral Care and Counseling, Yale Divinity School, New Haven, CT (E-mail: ksamuel.lee@yale.edu).

[Haworth co-indexing entry note]: "Toward Multicultural Competencies for Pastoral/Spiritual Care Providers in Clinical Settings: Response to Anderson, Fukuyama, and Sevig." Lee, K. Samuel. Co-published simultaneously in *Journal of Health Care Chaplaincy* (The Haworth Pastoral Press, an imprint of The Haworth Press, Inc.) Vol. 13, No. 2, 2004, pp. 43-50; and: *Ministry in the Spiritual and Cultural Diversity of Health Care: Increasing the Competency of Chaplains* (ed: Robert G. Anderson, and Mary A. Fukuyama) The Haworth Pastoral Press, an imprint of The Haworth Press, Inc., 2004, pp. 43-50. Single or multiple copies of this article are available for a fee from The Haworth Document Delivery Service [1-800-HAWORTH, 9:00 a.m. - 5:00 p.m. (EST). E-mail address: docdelivery@haworthpress.com].

Digital Object Identifier: 10.1300/J080v13n02_03

KEYWORDS. Multicultural chaplaincy, religion, spirituality

A "multicultural revolution" that challenges the traditional health care delivery system (Sue, Bingham, Porché-Burke, and Vasquez, 1999) has been taking place in the United States in recent decades. In response, a number of organizations related to health care delivery developed guidelines for multicultural competencies to better serve the increasingly diverse U.S. population (e.g., American Psychological Association, 2003; National Association of Social Workers, 2001; U.S. Department of Health and Human Services, 2001). Various organizations of health care chaplaincy, too, have been responding by considering multicultural competencies for their organizations. The Association for Clinical Pastoral Education (ACPE) created the Multicultural Competencies Task Force in 2001, and the task force has been working on a proposal to include multicultural competencies in the ACPE's training and operation manuals. The *Journal of Supervision and Training in Ministry* published a special symposium on the topic of multicultural pastoral practice in clinical settings (DeVelder, Lee, and Griesel, 2002). This issue of the *Journal of Health Care Chaplaincy* is another example of how organizations related to health care chaplaincy are responding to the multicultural revolution in the United States.

As a result of a multicultural revolution in the U.S. that encompasses increased religious diversity, many chaplains have seen the need to change the name of their departments from "pastoral care" to "spiritual care." This is in recognition that "pastoral care" is distinctively Christian and excludes care provided by and for non-Christians. Despite the debate about the new terminology that will undoubtedly continue (e.g., Miller, Lawrence, and Powell, 2003), the need to study "spirituality" in the psychological practices has been widely recognized and has resulted in many publications by psychologists since the 1990s. Such a change is expected to impact the fields of pastoral care, pastoral theology, and the ways seminary professors conceive of these traditional fields.

Elena Cohen (1999) of the Center for Child Health and Mental Health Policy enumerates the reasons for multicultural competencies in health care practices. They are (1) "to respond to current and projected demographic changes in the United States," (2) "to eliminate long-standing disparities in the health status of people of diverse racial, ethnic, and cultural backgrounds," (3) "to meet legislative, regulatory, and accreditation mandates," and (4) "to gain a competitive edge in the market place." In addition to Cohen's rationale, pastoral or spiritual care providers must cultivate theological understanding that is born out of their religious tradition because what sets pastoral or spiritual practice apart from other clinical and psychological practices is that very theological identity. Adoption of multicultural competencies that promote attitudinal-cognitive-behavioral learning must be complemented by theological rationale to serve pastoral practitioners adequately in the long run.

Considering a theological foundation in multicultural pastoral practice portends enormous challenge. It does so because constructs used in theology and psychology are categorically distinct, although they may share common features. For example, when a psychologist (e.g., Steinberg, 1986) considers the meaning of love between couples, he sees a triangle of love that consists of passion, intimacy, and commitment and evolves through the life span. When a feminist pastoral theologian (Miller-McLemore, at press) considers the meaning of love between couples, she sees two sides of a coin held in tension between mutuality and self-giving. Also consider Fukuyama and Sevig's comparing of spiritual and multicultural values. I wonder whether we can really "compare" the so-called spiritual values of "grace, intimacy, creativity" to the so-called multicultural values of "commitment and humor"? Such comparison, in my opinion, results in unnecessary and unfruitful syncretism of psychology and theology that ignores the distinctiveness and integrity of both disciplines.

Undoubtedly, much work must be done to explain the interplay between psychology and theology. To that end, Joann Wolski Conn (1985) examines the differential underlying premises, though somewhat reductionistically, of theology and psychology by contrasting Christian spirituality and psychological maturity. She shows various ways that theology and psychology may (or may not) come together.

She proposes that both theology and psychology must learn from each other to more fully construct human experience.

In a more specific way, William Doherty (1999) recognizes that there are "three domains of language and meaning" in clinical practice, including the domains of "the clinical world of mental health, the moral realm of obligations, and the spiritual realm of transcendent meaning." He compares these three domains to Don Browning's (1987) "ultimate metaphors (theology), obligation (ethics), and psychology," which Browning considers to be categorically distinct. These domains overlap each other but must remain distinct "for purposes of clarity" as well as their own integrity. Perhaps more helpful than Fukuyama and Sevig's comparison of spiritual and multicultural values, Doherty's model presents three domains of language and meaning as described in Figure 1.

If Browning and Doherty are correct in assuming that the three domains described in Figure 1 are categorically distinct, what are the implications for developing multicultural competencies in pastoral or spiritual practice in clinical settings? I propose that three domains of language and meaning be seriously considered: theological, ethical, and clinical. Because most multicultural competency guidelines address the ethical and clinical domains, I shall limit myself in providing some examples of what I consider the essential theological issues.

In cultivating multicultural chaplains who are theologically grounded, we need to consider the call to serve the culturally different (cf. Jonah in Nineveh, the Good Samaritan story, Jesus' ministry with the Syro-Phoenician woman or the woman at Jacob's Well). The traditional religious understanding of the call, in my opinion, is better than Fukuyama and Sevig's term such as "passion." Theological consideration should also include the chaplain's ability to engage in multicultural hermeneutics of texts that are considered authoritative within his or her religious tradition. This recognizes that often the multicultural *context* in which the chaplain finds himself or herself shapes how the *text* is to be read. For example, in considering that the event of Exodus is not exclusively for the slave Jews in Egypt, Brueggemann (1998) considers the meaning of "Exodus in the plural" in the Hebrew scripture. Brueggemann illustrates how a multiculturally competent biblical scholar should read the He-

FIGURE 1. Three Domains of Language and Meaning

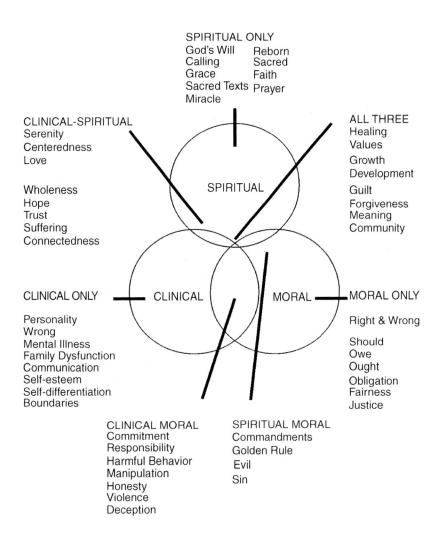

Note: Figure 1 adapted from: Dougherty, p. 185.

brew scripture to be inclusive of God's salvation. If, however, the chaplain is lost within his or her own ethnocentric theological perspective or worldview and cannot consider the *local context* (Schreiter, 1985) of patients, his or her hermeneutics may result in dogmatic imposition, cultural imperialism, or cultural violence. The ability to engage in interreligious dialogue is another component that should be included in the theological consideration of multicultural competencies. All in all, the basic theological foundation of multicultural competencies must show how *who we are theologically shapes what we do* as pastoral or spiritual care providers in clinical settings.

The cultural and religious diversity addressed by Fukuyama and Sevig and by Anderson in this volume clearly points to the urgency to develop multicultural competencies to better serve the culturally diverse clientele. Consequently, their emphasis is naturally placed on the chaplain-in-practice who is faced with the culturally different client. Multicultural competencies, however, must be reflected in all aspects of health care chaplaincy, not only in service delivery but also in recruitment and teaching of chaplains-to-be as well as in the ways training centers do their business. This point has been widely advocated (Sue et al., 1999; also see Sue et al., 1998).

A glimpse of cultural diversity among chaplain trainees can be seen in a snapshot survey of CPE students done by the ACPE during the summer of 2002. There were 2,050 CPE students during the summer of 2002, out of which 528 students returned the survey. My analyses of the data showed a tremendous range of diversity among them. Students were evenly divided by sex (52.3% female and 47.7% male). Students' ages ranged from 22 to 65 years. At least 48 denominations were represented, including Judaism and Buddhism. Twelve persons reported some physical and mental handicapping conditions. Out of 112 ethnic minority students, 5.5 percent were African American, 0.6 percent described themselves as Asian American, 2.1 percent were Hispanic American, 0.8 percent reported being Native American, and 9.7 percent were international students. International students came from Australia, Bolivia, Brazil, Canada, China, Columbia, India, England, Ethiopia, Germany, Haiti, Israel, Japan, Kenya, Korea, Mexico, Myanmar, Netherlands, Nigeria, Norway, Palestine, Peru, Philippines, South Africa, Taiwan, Tanzania, Uganda, Uruguay, Venezuela, Vietnam, and Zambia.

The cultural diversity that CPE students bring to their training sites is mind-boggling. In view of this diversity of chaplains-to-be, one cannot help but ask: Who is training this diverse group of chaplains-to-be today? This is a poignant question when we consider that today's health care chaplaincy organizations predominantly consist of European American chaplains. Multicultural competency guidelines, therefore, must address how clinical centers can become multiculturally transformed and how they can help their predominantly European American chaplain trainers become more multiculturally competent. Such consideration points to the necessity to include in these guidelines how the training centers can recruit more culturally different chaplains so that the centers may more closely reflect the one-third of the U.S. population that are non-white European Americans. Clearly, we have a long way to go, but it is a worthwhile journey to take because, in becoming multicultural, we will all learn a lot more about who we are and who we can become.

AUTHOR NOTE

K. Samuel Lee is Visiting Assistant Professor of Pastoral Care and Counseling at Yale University Divinity School. His research interests focus on multicultural pastoral care, counseling, and pastoral theology. He has written numerous articles on multicultural theological education and multicultural competencies in clinical pastoral practice, and has contributed articles on the Korean American Church. He is an ordained minister in the United Methodist Church. From 1995 to 2002 he served as the Associate Dean and Assistant Professor of Pastoral Care and Theology at Wesley Theological Seminary. He is currently the Steering Committee Chairperson of the Society for Pastoral Theology and a member of the Multicultural Competencies Task Force of the Association of Clinical Pastoral Education. He received his MDiv from Yale University and PhD in counseling psychology from Arizona State University.

REFERENCES

American Psychological Association. (2003). Guidelines on multicultural education, training, research, practice, and organizational change for psychologists. *American Psychologist*, 58(5), 377-402. Also available at *http://www.apa.org/pi/multiculturalguidelines.pdf*.

Browning, D. (1987). *Religious thought and the modern psychologies*. Philadelphia Fortress Press.

Brueggemann, W. (1998). "Exodus" in the plural (Amos 9:7). In Brueggemann, W., & Stroup, G. (Eds.) *Many voices one God: Being faithful in a pluralistic world*, (pp. 15-34). Louisville: Westminster John Knox Press.

Cohen, E. (1999). Policy brief 1: National Center for Cultural Competency, winter 1999, *Georgetown University Child Development Center*, pp. 2-7.

Conn, J.W. (1985). Spirituality and personal maturity. In Wicks, R., Parsons, R., & Capps, D. (Eds.) *Clinical handbook of pastoral counseling volume 1 expanded edition*, (pp. 37-57). NY: Integration Books.

DeVelder, J. Lee, K.S., & Griesel, A. (Eds.) (2002). Symposium: Multiculturality in the student-supervisor/teacher relationship. *Journal of Supervision and Training in Ministry*. 22.

Doherty, W. (1999). Morality and spirituality in therapy. In Walsh, F. (Ed.) *Spiritual resources in family therapy* (pp. 179-192). NY: Guilford Press.

Miller, R., Lawrence, R., & Powell, R. (2003). Guest editorial. *Journal of Pastoral Care and Counseling*, 57(2), 111-116.

Miller-McLemore, B. (2003 at press). Sloppy mutuality: Love and justice for children and adults. In Anderson, H., Miller-McLemore, B., Foley, E., & Schreiter, R. (Eds.), *Mutuality Matters: The Promise and Peril of Democratic Families*. Chicago: Sheed & Ward.

National Association of Social Workers. (2001). *NASW standards for cultural competency in social work practice (brochure)*. NASW Press.

Schreiter, R. (1997). Constructing local theologies. NY: Orbis Books.

Sternberg R. (1986). A triangular theory of love. *Psychological Review*, 93, 119-135.

Sue, D.W., Bingham, R. P, Porché-Burke, L., & Vasquez, M. (1999). The diversification of psychology: A multicultural revolution. *American Psychologist*, 54(12), 1061-1069.

Sue, D.W., Carter, R.T., Casas, J. M., Fouad, N.A., Ivey, A.E., Jensen, M., LaFromboise, T., Manese, J.E., Ponterotto, J.G., & Vazquez-Nutall, E. (1998). *Multicultural counseling competencies: Individual and organizational development*. Thousand Oaks, CA: Sage Publications.

U.S. Department of Health and Human Services. (March, 2001). National standards for culturally and linguistically appropriate services in health care: Final report.

Forging Spiritual and Cultural Competency in Spiritual Care-Givers: A Response to Fukuyama and Sevig and Anderson

Marsha Wiggins Frame, PhD

KEYWORDS. Multicultural chaplaincy, religion, spirituality

In their articles, Anderson and then Fukuyama and Sevig make convincing cases for the need for health care chaplains to become competent in spiritual and cultural diversity. As a United Methodist clergywoman for nearly 30 years, and as a counselor educator for the past 10 years, I

Marsha Wiggins Frame is Associate Professor and Chair of Counseling Psychology and Counselor Education, University of Colorado at Denver, Denver, CO (E-mail: mframe@ceo.cudenver.edu).

[Haworth co-indexing entry note]: "Forging Spiritual and Cultural Competency in Spiritual Care-Givers: A Response to Fukuyama and Sevig and Anderson." Frame, Marsha Wiggins. Co-published simultaneously in *Journal of Health Care Chaplaincy* (The Haworth Pastoral Press, an imprint of The Haworth Press, Inc.) Vol. 13, No. 2, 2004, pp. 51-58; and: *Ministry in the Spiritual and Cultural Diversity of Health Care: Increasing the Competency of Chaplains* (ed: Robert G. Anderson, and Mary A. Fukuyama) The Haworth Pastoral Press, an imprint of The Haworth Press, Inc., 2004, pp. 51-58. Single or multiple copies of this article are available for a fee from The Haworth Document Delivery Service [1-800-HAWORTH, 9:00 a.m. - 5:00 p.m. (EST). E-mail address: docdelivery@haworthpress.com].

http://www.haworthpress.com/web/JHCC
Digital Object Identifier: 10.1300/J080v13n02_04

applaud the intersection of spiritual and cultural diversity with pastoral care.

Anderson's five dimensions of spiritual and cultural competency are a useful beginning for the journey toward chaplains being equipped to provide pastoral care to a variety of persons from a wide range of religious, spiritual, and cultural contexts. The cases he provides illustrate well the complex web in which chaplains often find themselves.

Fukuyama and Sevig are accurate when they speak of spirituality and religion being embedded in culture, and in their careful descriptions of cultural diversity and delineation of the distinctions between religion and spirituality. The themes in their article parallel closely my own work (Frame, 2003). In response to Anderson's steps and Fukuyama and Sevig's key points on the journey, I offer specific strategies and tools that may assist chaplains in acquiring spiritual and cultural competency.

SELF-AWARENESS

One of the strengths of clinical pastoral education (CPE) is experiential learning with its emphasis on integrating cognitive and emotional aspects of training with theological reflection. Thus, issues related to the self-of-the-chaplain are prominent. Becoming competent in working with persons from diverse spiritual, racial, ethnic, and cultural backgrounds requires intensive self-reflection. Indeed, competency in this arena is predicated on spiritual care providers' confronting their own racism and their religious/spiritual biases. Essentially, this process is akin to repentance in that it involves practicing *metanoia*, that is, turning around and going a new way. For Caucasians, confronting racism involves challenging the ways that they consciously or unconsciously maintain the attitude that people of color are inferior or that these groups' differences are unacceptable (Batts, 1998). For people of color, it means acknowledging internalized racism and the self-deprecation that may accompany it. Addressing religious/spiritual bias involves examining ways in which spiritual care providers may use their own religious or spiritual worldview as the standard against which all others are measured. It means giving up the notion that our beliefs and practices are the only path to the divine. Moreover, coming to terms with oneself and one's own spiritual and cultural web requires recognizing the ways in which being a member of the dominant culture confers power and privilege that is not available to marginalized groups. For example, when White professionals of either gender enter a hospital or other health care setting, they are less likely to be viewed with suspicion than their counterparts who are people of color. When representatives of Judeo-Christian religious groups practice their faith in public, usually they are not seen as peculiar or heretical. Thus, power and privilege operate to exclude and penalize those who are in the minority in terms of race, ethnicity, culture or spiritual perspective.

Knowing one's own spiritual and cultural set suggests the need for chaplains of all cultural groups and religious/spiritual worldviews to claim their heritage and the values associated with it. For people of color, this assignment may be accomplished more easily than for Whites because the latter often believe they have no particular culture or ethnicity-that these terms apply only to people of color (Giordano & McGoldrick, 1996). One way of getting in touch with one's cultural and religious/spiritual history is for seasoned chaplains as well as those in training to create cultural (Hardy & Laszloffy, 1995) and spiritual (Frame, 2001) genograms. These family maps provide graphic illustrations of the cultural and spiritual roots and patterns that impact individuals and families. They also serve as excellent learning tools about multicultural and multispiritual functioning. Through building cultural and spiritual genograms, participants attain visceral self-awareness of who they are and the myriad of influences that have shaped them. This broadened perspective is a critical step in achieving multicultural and multispiritual competency.

The importance of acknowledging the limitations of one's competency and seeking assistance should not be overlooked. Such awareness does not come without a struggle that demands deep introspection, firm accountability, and on-going emotional support. Being aware of one's limits often results in the necessity for spiritual caregivers to seek assistance from others skilled in working within a particular cultural, ethnic or religious community.

KNOWLEDGE OF OTHERNESS

Another aspect of becoming competent in spiritual and cultural realities involves the ability to learn about and embrace difference. Part of this learning is didactic and cognitive. It requires reading and research to gain information about races, cultures, religions, and spirituality different from one's own. Helms and Cook in their book, *Using Race and Culture in Counseling and Psychotherapy (1999)* describe the sociopolitical histories of various racial and ethnic groups and provide exercises whereby readers can become more culture-sensitive. McGoldrick, Giordano, and Pearce (1996) in their edited volume, *Ethnicity and Family Therapy* provide a wealth of information about a wide range of ethnic groups' values, beliefs, practices, and how they respond to psychological interventions. Richards and Bergin (2000) discuss the religious and spiritual belief systems of Christian, Eastern, and Ethnic spiritualities and assist psychotherapists and spiritual care givers in working with these populations. Amassing literature and gathering facts, however, is not sufficient. Learning about difference must also be experiential. It involves cultivating relationships with persons of divergent religions, races, ethnicities, and cultures. It means intentionally immersing oneself in the festivals, rituals, celebrations, and routines of those who hail from different traditions from our own. Learning about difference experientially means attending conferences and gatherings sponsored by racial, ethnic, religious, and cultural groups that are unfamiliar to us and by so doing beginning to be able to take another perspective.

SKILL ACQUISITION

Being competent to address religious/spiritual and cultural diversity requires not just self-awareness and knowledge, but the ability to act professionally and communicate effectively with persons different from ourselves. For example, many spiritual care givers and counselors have been trained in attending behaviors including minimal encouragers (MmHumm) and reflections of feelings. However, these communication styles either may not exist in nonwhite cultures or may feel ingenuine (Helms & Cook, 1999). In addition, some caregivers use a nondirective communication style when some patients might prefer more directive approaches (Borrego, Chavez, & Titley, 1982). Language, too, may create communication difficulties. When English is a patient's second language, she or he may resort to "language switching" (Helms & Cook, 1999, p. 193) in a crisis. That is, the patient may need to speak in his or her first language to be delivered from the stress-related paralysis of being caught between two languages. Chaplains who encourage clients to speak their first language and later translate facilitate communication across cultural differences. Likewise, patients who engage in glossolalia (speaking in tongues) during spiritual ecstasy may need to be encouraged to express themselves and then interpret for the chaplain if this practice is not within his or her tradition. In these ways, spiritual care givers may pay attention to communication styles attributed to different cultures or spiritual practices.

ASSESSING BARRIERS

Regardless of spiritual care providers' and patients' backgrounds, often there will be contextual and relational barriers that must be noted and addressed. Social and economic class, position of power in the institution or the society, gender, sexual orientation, physical, and mental ability and other differences can be viewed as barriers to providing pastoral care to patients and their families. Such obstacles may create issues of trust in both the spiritual care provider and the recipients of that care. At times, it may be appropriate to address the discomfort concerning difference with patients and their families. Open acknowledgement frequently is the first step toward improved communication and mutual understanding.

WILLINGNESS TO LEARN

Certainly an attitude of openness and receptivity is a prerequisite for success in multispiritual/cultural interaction. Care-givers' genuine respect for difference can create a "transitional zone" between comfort and discomfort. However, I disagree with Anderson (this volume) regarding the strategy of inviting the patient to "teach him [the chaplain] more about valued traditions and beliefs." It seems to me that it is the duty of the chaplain to learn about cultural and religious difference in another setting and not to place that burden on his patient. Indeed, Arredondo et al. (1996) state specifically that one strategy for becoming more multiculturally competent is to "accept that it is your responsibility to learn about other cultures and implications in counseling and not to expect or rely on individuals from those cultures to teach you" (p. 24). Moreover, it is extremely tiring and an energy drain when patients and other care recipients must shoulder the burden of educating persons of other cultures about themselves. Such an obligation becomes an albatross and a hindrance to cultural competency. Instead, seeking support from others from one's own culture who also are learning can be helpful. In addition, engaging a mentor from another culture who is also working on multicultural/spiritual competency is useful for reciprocal benefits (Arrendondo et al., 1996). Consulting with professionals from cultures and religious/spiritual traditions different from one's own, especially indigenous healers, can expand competency in these areas (Helms & Cook, 1999). For example, curanderos in Mexican culture are folk healers who are trusted for assistance with maladies that have psychological components (Falicov, 1996). American Indian traditional healers use spiritual legends and practices to bring patients into harmony with their environment (LaFromboise, 1988). The Asian Indian tradition of Ayurveda relies on the unity of body, mind, and spirit (Das, 1987). Collaboration with such healers may bring about wholeness for patients and families undergoing the stress of an illness.

In conclusion, Anderson, and Fukuyama and Sevig, have sounded the call for spiritual care providers to take seriously the need to become competent when working with patients and others from different backgrounds and traditions. The challenge, then, is to be intentional about gaining self-awareness, knowledge, and skills to increase culturally and spiritually effective practice. This work involves diligent and often painful self-reflection, active engagement with disparate worldviews, willingness to suspend one's need to be right or to function as an expert, consultation and supervision with skilled trainers and mentors, and most of all, a commitment to change. The invitation has been extended. Who will respond?

AUTHOR NOTE

Marsha Wiggins Frame is Associate Professor and Chair of Counseling Psychology and Counselor Education at the University of Colorado at Denver. She is also an ordained United Methodist minister and has served churches in the Florida Conference for over 13 years. Her research interest lies in the intersection of spirituality and counseling. Recently, she published a textbook on this topic entitled, Integrating Religion and Spirituality into Counseling: A Comprehensive Approach.

REFERENCES

Arredondo, P., Toporek, R., Brown, S., Jones, J., Lock, D. C., Sanchez, J., & Stadler, H. (1996). *Operationalization of the multicultural counseling competencies. Alexandria, VA: American Counseling Association.*

Batts, V. (1998). Modern racism: New melody for the same old tunes. Visions Training Manual. Arlington, MA: Author.

Borrego, R. L., Chavez, E. L., & Titley, R. W. (1982). Effect of counselor technique on Mexican-American and Anglo-American self-disclosure and counselor perception. *Journal of Counseling Psychology, 29,* 538-541.

Das, A. K. (1987). Indigenous models of therapy in traditional Asian societies. *Journal of Multicultural Counseling and Development, 15*, 25-37.

Falicov, C. J. (1996). Mexican families. In M. McGoldrick, J. Giordano, & J. K. Pearce (Eds.), *Ethnicity and family therapy* (2nd ed). (pp. 169-182). New York: Guilford.

Frame, M. W. (2003). Integrating religion and spirituality into counseling: A comprehensive approach. Pacific Grove, CA: Brooks/Cole.

Frame, M. W. (2001). The spiritual genogram in training and supervision. *The Family Journal, 9*, 109-115.

Giordano, J., & McGoldrick, M. (1996). European Families: An overview. In M. McGoldrick, J. Giordano, & J. K. Pearce (Eds.), *Ethnicity and family therapy* (2nd ed). (pp. 427-441). New York: Guilford.

Hardy, K. V., & Laszoffy, T. A. (1995). The cultural genogram: Key to training culturally competent family therapists. *Journal of Martial and Family Therapy, 21*, 227-237.

Helms, J. E., & Cook, D. A. (1999). *Using race and culture in counseling and psychotherapy*. Needham Heights, MA: Allyn & Bacon.

LaFromboise, T. D. (1988). American Indian mental health policy. *American Psychologist, 43*, 388-397.

McGoldrick, M., Giordano, J., & Pearce, J. K. (Eds.), (1996). *Ethnicity and family therapy* (2nd ed). New York: Guilford.

Richards, P. S., & Bergin, A. E. (2000). *Handbook of psychotherapy and religious diversity*. Washington, D.C.: American Psychological Association.

Definitions, Obstacles, and Standards of Care for the Integration of Spiritual and Cultural Competency Within Health Care Chaplaincy

Stephen W. Cook, PhD

KEYWORDS. Multicultural chaplaincy, religion, spirituality

The feature articles in this issue by Anderson (2004) and Fukuyama and Sevig (2004) provide helpful insight and point for consideration regarding the issues involved in nurturing a multicultural approach to the occupation of health care chaplaincy. My response to these articles will address definitional and standard of care issues, as well as discussing

---

Stephen W. Cook is affiliated with Texas Tech University, Lubbock, TX (E-mail: s.cook@ttu.edu).

[Haworth co-indexing entry note]: "Definitions, Obstacles, and Standards of Care for the Intergration of Spiritual and Cultural Competency Within Health Care Chaplaincy." Cook, Stephen W. Co-published simultaneously in *Journal of Health Care Chaplaincy* (The Haworth Pastoral Press, an imprint of The Haworth Press, Inc.) Vol. 13, No. 2, 2004, pp. 59-69; and: *Ministry in the Spiritual and Cultural Diversity of Health Care: Increasing the Competency of Chaplains* (ed: Robert G. Anderson, and Mary A. Fukuyama) The Haworth Pastoral Press, an imprint of The Haworth Press, Inc., 2004, pp. 59-69. Single or multiple copies of this article are available for a fee from The Haworth Document Delivery Service [1-800-HAWORTH, 9:00 a.m. - 5:00 p.m. (EST). E-mail address: docdelivery@haworthpress.com].

http://www.haworthpress.com/web/JHCC
Digital Object Identifier: 10.1300/J080v13n02_05

possible obstacles to fostering a genuine multicultural perspective among health care caregivers, particularly chaplains.

DEFINITIONS

The authors of both articles devote attention to definitions of religion and spirituality. In the psychology of religion, there has been much discussion about definitions and meanings of these two constructs (e.g., Cook, Borman, Moore, & Kunkel, 2000; Pargament, Sullivan, Balzer, Van Haitsma, & Raymark, 1995; Zinnbauer et al., 1997). Spirituality has only a recent history in professional psychology, but this term has become more accepted and, for many people, preferable to religion or religiousness for describing their experience (Spilka, Hood, Hunsberger, & Gorsuch, 2003). Thankfully, Fukuyama and Sevig did not provide definitions of religiousness and spirituality in such a way as to demonize religion and beatify spirituality (pardon the puns), such as has been the recent trend (Pargament, 1999). For the majority of people, both religion and spirituality coexist (e.g., Zinnbauer et al., 1997) and would seem to serve a meaningful function in their lives. Pargament (1999) argues that spirituality is rarely experienced without the context of religion, and that religion is seldom engaged without some acknowledgment of spirituality. Dotts, a medical ethicist, clergy, and senior vice president in a regional hospital, creates a wonderful word picture of how spirituality and religion interact-spirituality is the wine, which is held in the cup of religion (personal communication, September 5, 2003). For most people, although certainly not all, both religion and spirituality serve important roles and both are important for caregivers to assess.

In our recognition that spirituality can be expressed and experienced in a variety of ways, it is also important to draw boundaries about what is distinctive about religion and spirituality–i.e., what distinguishes religion/spirituality from a philosophy of life, one's morals, an ethical code, etc. Care should be taken that the uniqueness of religiousness and spirituality doesn't get lost among efforts to embrace multiple spiritual perspectives. Certainly the door can be opened wider in many health care settings in terms of accepting more diverse spiritual perspectives of patients. However, I am concerned that some definitions of religion and particularly spirituality can become so broad as to lose the distinctiveness that they possess apart from other sources of meaning and standards for living. Spirituality and religion are distinguished by some sense or acknowledgment of "the sacred" (Pargament, 1997); others (e.g., Plante & Sherman, 2001) distinguish them by referring to the "transcendent."

On a related note, I caution against blurring the distinctions between cultural and spiritual competence, as Anderson seemed to imply. Similarly to Fukuyama and Sevig, I conceive that culture is a broader construct that includes a variety of components such as ethnicity, socioeconomic status, gender, sexual orientation, etc., in addition to spirituality. Spirituality is one of many elements that comprise our cultural identity.

POSSIBLE OBSTACLES TO INCORPORATING MULTICULTURALISM AND INTERFAITH PERSPECTIVES

Considering the previously described definitional issues, however, seems more like an academic exercise compared to dealing with the difficulty of actively working with spiritual issues from a true multicultural perspective as a diverse group of health care professionals or caregivers. Caregivers may be able to work with patients of different spiritual orientations by helping patients see how well their life fits with their identified orientation. However, Anderson hit upon a critical issue when he asked, "Does my worldview allow for pluralistic reality"? More specifically, what happens if chaplains have a spiritual perspective that sees their way as the only true way–i.e., does not see other spiritual paths as legitimate or at least not as valid as their own spiritual path? Can chaplains genuinely appreciate and value others given this perspective? Can only chaplains who truly value the total diversity of spiritual perspectives be those who have a universalist approach? I wonder how someone who advocates for a spiritually inclusive approach can be truly tolerant and accepting of someone whose spiritual approach is not inclusive.

These questions were made more salient to me last week after we held a daylong conference on spirituality and health care. A member of the local Christian clergy asked me what kind of response a caregiver can have to patients of different spiritual orientations when the caregiver believes their spiritual orientation provides the only path to God. I could not come up with a good response to this. Can one truly "set aside" one's cultural set or web of meaning? (Cf. Anderson's discussion). I believe that our own cultural web of meaning, including our religious/spiritual orientation, will always be present in our interactions with patients to some degree, whether implicit or explicit. I suggest that it would be more helpful to recognize how our own spiritual perspective affects our interactions with patients in order to more effectively care for others with whom we relate.

In a related vein, could there be something unique in the growth that can be fostered between a chaplain and a patient who have different spiritual orientations? Perhaps it might help people to step outside their own belief system occasionally in order to more accurately examine our own spiritual perspective and engender spiritual growth. Sometimes caregivers and particularly educators of caregivers assume that the more informed a caregiver is about a patient's spiritual perspective, the better. However, don't forget that caregivers have particular expertise from their professional training and also potentially from their own, perhaps different, spiritual perspectives. People who spend time more exclusively within their own religious community, might find alternate perspectives helpful, albeit threatening to their existing spiritual orientation.

Both feature articles included recognition that a western Judeo-Christian individualistic perspective or bias of individualism is present in many health-care professionals in the United States. Caregivers need to be mindful about tailoring interventions to more closely fit the needs and preferences of patients from more collectivist cultures–e.g., involving family members and other members of a patient's cultural group in the treatment process. I also believe that the predominant emphasis on quick diagnosis and problem-focused, specialized intervention, which is central to the medical model, often runs counter to efforts to foster a true multicultural perspective among health care professionals. A multicultural perspective is fostered by a hesitancy to rush to conclusions, careful listening to the client's narrative, and the withholding of premature formulations and patient conceptualizations, which might be unduly influenced by the caregiver more than by the patient. Taking time to understand any individual's spiritual orientation, even when the spiritual orientation of the chaplain and the patient fall within the same general tradition, seems crucial when working toward a goal of cultural competency.

When further considering how ideas outlined in the feature articles could best be put into practice, I wondered when Fukuyama and Sevig discussed the multicultural learning processes of Hoopes (1979) and their own OTAID model, if these developmental models would be valid for someone who comes from more conservative religious/spiritual traditions. For instance, I wonder if leaders or experts within some spiritual orientations– i.e., those leaders assumed to be more mature in their spiritual orientation– would agree that these models are valid if they believe that their spiritual path, as I alluded to earlier, is the only valid direction for growth. Similarly, I question whether some religious/spiritual leaders/experts would agree that people have a "spiritual connection with all living beings" as Fukuyama and Sevig argue in this volume. In other words, I wrestle with the idea that any model of religious or spiritual developmental can be developed which would be valid for all spiritual orientations, much less even for all the various denominations within one particular spiritual orientation. For example, can a model of spiritual development or spiritual maturity be accurate for both Sunni and Shiite Muslims?

STANDARDS OF CARE

I appreciate Fukuyama and Sevig's caveat that value conflicts may create ethical problems for caregivers. I certainly believe that when caregivers find that they cannot provide good care to a patient or may harm a patient, it is best to refer. However, this brings up two difficult issues. First of all, might different people, and people from different spiritual orientations, define "good care" differently? How is "good care" operationalized? Pargament (1997, chap. 10) tackled this difficult question in the context of evaluating outcomes of religious coping, Not only does he review evidence regarding how people generally appraise the utility of their own religious coping efforts, but he also explores how religious coping is linked to more objective measures of outcome. Pargament (1997) notes, "It is important to consider how religious coping impacts on the full range of human functioning-physical, social, psychological, and spiritual" (p. 313). For instance, Fukuyama and Sevig in their article refer to the contentious issue of abortion. Obviously pro-choice and pro-life advocates might differ on what they see as "good care" in many situations for a pregnant woman considering abortion. Many times what may seem harmful mentally, emotionally, and physically is seen by a patient as helpful for their spiritual welfare. Caregivers need to be cognizant of this and respect this, but maybe there is a point when caregivers will want to draw the line in terms of being nonjudgmental about a patient's beliefs and behaviors.

For instance, consider how a chaplain could respond to someone who refuses medical treatments deemed crucial by physicians to their child (which is similar to Anderson's second case study). Can or should chaplains respond with an attitude of neutrality to this issue? There are many situations in which patients struggle with balancing physical or psychological concerns with spiritual concerns–e.g., dealing with end-of-life issues. In such circumstances it may be easy to see this problem in all or nothing terms–e.g., either the mother's wishes for spiritual healing are respected and the child is given no medical treatment, or the child receives medical treatment while the mother's spiritual concerns are dismissed. However, it is often helpful to seek ways in which alternate courses of actions can be offered. For instance, in this example medical treatment could occur alongside the mother's efforts toward spiritual healing for the child.

A second issue that should be considered, assuming that caregivers decide that they cannot provide good care to a patient, is how the corresponding referral can best be conducted. Caregiver should consider what implicit and explicit messages will be conveyed by the referral. For instance, caregivers may implicitly convey that the patient is being referred because of a spiritual orientation that is considered wrong or unacceptable. Caregivers should take care when referring so that their communications do not become manipulative or judgmental.

Another quality of care concern is the importance of conducting a careful and comprehensive assessment of how a patient's spiritual "web of meaning" (as described by Anderson) impacts her/his life. Anderson referred to Allport's intrinsic and extrinsic religiousness (Allport & Ross, 1967), which is useful for assessment purposes. For example, to what extent does a patient's spirituality/religion serve as a means to an end (extrinsic religiousness), and to what extent does it serve as end in itself (intrinsic religiousness). This can be highly relevant, particularly in healthcare settings when assessing the extent to which a client's spirituality, combined with other aspects of his/her culture, serves as a resource for healing. To what extent is pain and suffering seen as a consequence of life events or spiritual health, and to what extent is pain and suffering seen as a path toward spiritual growth? Hill and Hood (1999) describe a plethora of pencil and paper measures that can aid caregivers in their assessment.

After time is spent carefully assessing a patient's spirituality, what happens when caregivers truly believe that someone has unhealthy attitudes or behaviors that seem to emanate primarily from her/his spiritual/religious orientation? Do caregivers challenge the patient's beliefs or confront the patient about these unhealthy aspects of spirituality? Should only a leader within their spiritual orientation challenge these beliefs? Particularly in these situations caregivers should consult with leaders/experts from the client's spiritual orientation. Anderson mentioned the importance of consultation in his article. Health care professionals often stress the importance of consultation, but it is easier said than done. For consultation to be successful, caregivers should make every effort to establish consistent meetings with peers who can serve as consultants for practice. Obviously, having a group of trusted peers serving as consultants from a wide variety of spiritual and other cultural perspectives is particularly helpful. For instance, if no one on a hospital chaplaincy's staff is very familiar with Native American spiritual traditions, it would be helpful to know who can be consulted when someone with this spiritual perspective is seeking services.

ENDING COMMENTS

I appreciated Fukuyama and Sevig's suggestions about balancing attempts to grow in the areas of multicultural understanding with efforts to nurture one's self. Productive personal work toward a greater understanding, awareness, and action in the area of multiculturalism takes a toll and often is difficult. As with other areas in our lives, we should balance our work on increasing our multicultural competency with occasional rest and renewal.

Both feature articles noted that to grow in our understanding of various cultural variables, it is helpful to experience life in different cultural environments. Perhaps programs in Clinical Pastoral Education could be offered (if not offered already) that provide chaplains an opportunity to be involved in this kind of real-life learning. Anderson noted that caretakers can also learn directly from the patients with whom they work. While this is very true, care should be taken when learning from others in this way. Some people from minority cultures might feel wary, minimized, or frustrated asked to educate their caregivers about their cultural perspective i.e., to be become teachers about their culture. It is the caregiver's responsibility to become knowledgeable of patients' cultural context, although many patients might be willing to cooperate in our efforts to become more knowledgeable about an unfamiliar culture.

I also agree that "spiritual qualities can assist the process of multi-culturalism" as Fukuyama and Sevig suggest in this volume. Many people who place a strong emphasis on the spiritual dimension in their lives are often quite open to seeking justice, pursuing social action, and showing compassion through their work with others. However, unfortunately it is clear that highly spiritual people can also engage in intolerance and abuse, refusing to accept others who are different. Caregivers need to be aware of the possible helpful as well as harmful roles that aspects of spirituality can plan in people's lives.

Finally, both feature articles mentioned issues of power and privilege, which are central to understanding multicultural issues. For instance, Fukuyama and Sevig noted "questioning and analyzing power is an underlying theme in multicultural work." It would be helpful to examine more closely how issues of power and privilege are manifested in the various treatment settings in which chaplains work. A critical examination of power/privilege issues within the health care system, particularly in terms of how they impact chaplains and the services chaplains provide, would be particularly useful. For instance, what would happen if someone who was promoted to be the head administrator of chaplaincy services in a large hospital possessed a spiritual orientation that was very different from the spiritual orientation traditionally practiced among chaplains in this hospital? Systemically, how could such a change in administration and in the dynamics of power be effectively managed? More generally, how might conflict be manifested and resolved in different organizations with varying spiritual and diverse cultural perspectives?

Overall, the call for the recognition and incorporation of spiritual and cultural competency among health care chaplains is worthwhile and critical to the growth of this profession, as most areas in our country tend to experience ever-increasing cultural diversity. Chaplains, as well as clinical pastoral education programs and health care administrators, need to work toward providing resources and establishing structures that will facilitate these skills for caregivers in the future.

AUTHOR NOTE

Stephen Cook is a psychologist, employed primarily as a faculty member in a psychology department where he serves as director for a counseling psychology PhD training program. One of his areas of specialization is exploring the relations between religion/spirituality and health. He maintains a very small independent practice where he conducts psychotherapy with adult individuals and couples; recently he was the consulting psychologist for a cardiac rehabilitation program in the largest area hospital. While he has lived in other parts of the United States, he was raised and currently lives in West Texas. He represents many aspects of cultural majority for the region–white, heterosexual, able-bodied, upper middle class, male, and claims Christianity as his religious affiliation. When considering the integration of a multicultural perspective in his own life, he admits that many times he is left with as many questions as answers. He has enjoyed the challenges of developing a multicultural perspective professionally as well as personally.

REFERENCES

Allport, G. W., & Ross, J. M. (1967). Personal religious orientation and prejudice. *Journal of Personality and Social Psychology, 5*, 432-443.

Anderson, R. G. (2004). The search for spiritual/cultural competencies in chaplaincy Practice: Five steps that mark the path. *Journal of Health Care Chaplaincy, 13*, 1-24.

Cook, S. W., Borman, P. D., Moore, M., & Kunkel, M. A. (2000). College students' perceptions of spiritual people and religious people. *Journal of Psychology and Theology, 28*, 125-137.

Fukuyama, M. A., & Sevig, T. D. (2004). Cultural diversity in pastoral care. *Journal of Health Care Chaplaincy, 13*, 25-41.

Hill, P.C., & Hood, R.W. (1999). *Measures of religiosity*. Birmingham, AL: Religious Education Press.

Hoopes, D.S. (1979). Intercultural communication concepts and the psychology of intercultural experience. In M.D. Pusch (Ed). *Multicultural education: A cross-cultural training approach*. LaGrange Park, IL: Intercultural Network, Inc.

Pargament, K. I. (1997). *The psychology of religion and coping*. New York: Guilford.

Pargament, K. I. (1999). *The psychology of religion and spirituality?* Yes and no. *International Journal for the Psychology of Religion, 9*, 3-16.

Pargament, K. I., Sullivan, M. S., Balzer, W. K., Van Haitsma, K. S., & Raymark, P. H. (1995). The many meanings of religiousness: A policy-capturing approach. *Journal of Personality, 63*, 953-983.

Plante, T. G., & Sherman, A. C. (2001). Research on faith and health: New approaches to old questions. In Plante, T. G., & Sherman, A. C. (Eds). *Faith and health: Psychological perspectives.* New York: Guilford.

Spilka, B., Hood, R. W., Jr., Hunsberger, B., & Gorsuch, R. (2003). *The psychology of religion: An empirical approach* (3rd ed.). New York: Guilford.

Zinnbauer, B. J., Pargament, K. I., Cole, B., Rye, M. S., Butter, E. M., Belavich, T. G., Hipp, K. M., Scott, A. B., & Kadar, J. L. (1997). Religion and spirituality: Unfuzzying the fuzzy. *Journal for the Scientific Study of Religion, 36,* 549-564.

The Chaplain's Path in Cultural
and Spiritual Sensitivity:
A Response
to Anderson, Fukuyama, and Sevig

Susan Koehne Wintz, MDiv, BCC

KEYWORDS. Multicultural chaplaincy, religion, spirituality

Professional chaplains, like all health care personnel, work within ever-changing environments. No longer can they simply assume an Anglo, Western, Judeo-Christian viewpoint. Patients, families, and healthcare workers likely differ from one another not only in ethnic and cultural backgrounds but also in their traditions, languages, and spiritual practices. Significant energy and focus is required to learn how to function

Susan Koehne Wintz is Staff Chaplain, St. Joseph's Hospital and Medical Center, Phoenix, AZ (E-mail: swintz@chw.edu).

[Haworth co-indexing entry note]: "The Chaplain's Path in Cultural and Spiritual Sensitivity: A Response to Anderson, Fukuyama, and Sevig ." Wintz, Susan Koehne. Co-published simultaneously in *Journal of Health Care Chaplaincy* (The Haworth Pastoral Press, an imprint of The Haworth Press, Inc.) Vol. 13, No. 2, 2004, pp. 71-82; and: *Ministry in the Spiritual and Cultural Diversity of Health Care: Increasing the Competency of Chaplains* (ed: Robert G. Anderson, and Mary A. Fukuyama) The Haworth Pastoral Press, an imprint of The Haworth Press, Inc., 2004, pp. 71-82. Single or multiple copies of this article are available for a fee from The Haworth Document Delivery Service [1-800-HAWORTH, 9:00 a.m. - 5:00 p.m. (EST). E-mail address: docdelivery@haworthpress.com].

http://www.haworthpress.com/web/JHCC
Digital Object Identifier: 10.1300/J080v13n02_06

within the demands imposed by these differences and healthcare organizations respond by providing education for their employees concerning cultural and spiritual differences.

One of the first statements that Fukuyama and Sevig make in their
contribution to this volume reads, "The question of how cultural diversity impacts the work of the healthcare chaplain is the focus of this article." My contribution here points out another important issue, namely
the question of how professional healthcare chaplains take leadership in
responding to cultural and spiritual diversity within healthcare environments.

CULTURAL SENSITIVITY IS INHERENT
IN THE CHAPLAIN'S PRACTICE

Within health care settings, chaplains are likely to be the most aware
of issues raised by the multicultural nature of the world, and influence
of those issues upon persons seeking health care. Clinical Pastoral Education (CPE), required by the largest chaplaincy certifying groups, focuses upon the process of chaplains becoming both personally and
professionally aware. The training, thought processes, and practices of
professionally certified chaplains emphasizes the importance of "doing
one's own work" concerning the issues raised by cultural and spiritual
differences. The call for competency is not new within the CPE movement or in the chaplaincy board certification process. In both, the emphasis is upon developing competency in various areas of learning
(CPE) and articulating that competency in the certification process.
What has been missing is the development of resources to demonstrate
ongoing competency by chaplains who have moved beyond their training and certification committees.

The question before us as chaplains, when dealing with any issue
including that of cultural competency, is how to make it applicable for our
own setting. The importance of continuing one's work around self-awareness and sensitivity issues cannot be over-emphasized. Again, this is not

new territory to clinically trained professional chaplains who understand the importance and rhythm of process. Attentiveness to cultural issues is certainly another process, and one that requires energy and intentional work. In this volume, Fukuyama, Sevig, and Anderson have skillfully acknowledged the importance of and some methods by which chaplains can work to achieve competency about cultural issues. These include the utilization of competency resources, peer review, and professional sharing of experiences-all examples of how one's work can be enhanced and improved.

However, these resources are not always easily available, especially to chaplains serving as sole staff members within departments geographically isolated from other professional chaplains. In addition, few if any resources on cultural competency available in the current market are applicable to the scope of practice of professional health care chaplains. Rather, they are directed towards nurses, physicians, or human resource specialists, omitting the spiritual component that is central to the chaplain's work. Even Fukuyama and Sevig themselves seem not to understand the unique scope of the chaplain, as they utilize primarily definitions from their own field of psychology rather than from professional spiritual care. In fact, they do not refer to pastoral care but rather to pastoral counseling, its cousin, which leads one to wonder if they are demonstrating the same kind of cultural unawareness that they advocate against.

Chaplain-oriented competency resources are needed. Wintz and Cooper developed "Cultural and Spiritual Sensitivity: A Learning Model" (2000) and its accompanying "Quick Guides for Cultures and Spiritual Traditions" (2000). These materials, the focus of a 2002 beta study by the Commission on Quality in Pastoral Services of the Association of Professional Chaplains (APC), provide resources by which chaplains can document their competency and also use as a teaching tool with clinical and medical staff within their organizations.

The materials begin by focusing on raising one's self-awareness through a series of activities that can be answered either individually or in a group setting. The questions invite learners to identify not only their personal traditions and beliefs, but also how they interact with others who are different. The importance of completing these self-awareness exercises is emphasized in order to set the stage for narrative learning materials.

The companion piece, "Quick Guides for Cultural and Spiritual Traditions" (2000), combines researched and new materials to provide a user-friendly resource for clinical staff. It is comprised of charts that cover various elements that may differ across cultural and spiritual traditions, inviting staff to begin conversations with patients, families, and/or one another about possible differences.

The materials, which can be found in the fall of 2003 on the Association of Professional Chaplains website *(www.professionalchaplains. org)*, are available for non-profit educational use. They are the first of a variety of resources and educational materials being developed by the organization for use by professional chaplains as competency and/or teaching tools.

In "Professional Chaplaincy: Its Role and Importance in Healthcare" (VandeCreek and Burton, 2001), a White Paper developed by a collaborative effort of five chaplaincy cognate groups, spirituality is described as "an awareness of relationships with all creation, an appreciation of presence and purpose that includes a sense of meaning." Chaplains work within an awareness of not only their own beliefs and practices that bring meaning into their lives, but also with knowledge of the importance of the spirituality of patients, families, and other members of the health care team. Many times chaplains serve as "cultural brokers" between patients or family and the hospital staff through the ways that they are able to identify cultural or spiritual issues of importance that arise and by bringing them to the forefront in the care plan. It is time that we become more assertive in claiming that role as a significant part of our professional scope of practice.

A SPIRITUAL PATHWAY FOR CULTURAL CHALLENGE

A clinical pathway is an interdisciplinary plan of best clinical practice for a specified group of patients, based on diagnostic criteria that have been studied and followed over time that aids the coordination and delivery of high quality care. A spiritual pathway, according to Hilsman (1998), is "a descriptive series of indicators of what may be happening to a person spiritually in the midst of a particular life predicament and some suggested ways of optimally assisting that person." Hilsman has identified several spiritual pathways (including prior grief, self neglect, family anxiety, patient fearfulness, and others) that describe particular patterns of patients' concerns. He advocates for chaplains to develop the skills needed to address those identified spiritual issues. He goes on to elaborate that spiritual pathways are composed of six elements including a name, a set of indicators, a set of actions, elements of optimal care, an outcome hoped for, a rationale on how addressing the particular issue will improve the health and satisfaction of the patient, and how it contributes to the mission of the particular care service.

Art Lucas, the director of chaplaincy at Barnes Jewish Hospital in St. Louis, created groundbreaking work in outcome-based spiritual care by developing the "Discipline for Pastoral Care Giving" (2001). The Discipline gives a framework for the chaplain's spiritual intervention and its integration into the total interdisciplinary plan of care. The Discipline begins by identifying the needs, hopes, and resources of the person for whom care is provided, which result in the development of a profile, including identified contributing outcomes, a plan, interventions, and a measurement of whether the outcomes were achieved during the encounter.

Both Hilsman's and Lucas' work can have a significant impact on the way in which chaplains approach their clinical care, including working with patients and families who are experiencing cultural challenges. Spiritual pathways can be developed, applied as appropriate, and used as teaching tools for chaplaincy students and clinical staff to demonstrate the outcomes resulting from the intervention of professional chaplains. Having an idea of what situations or issues might arise, how they are often expressed, and what spiritual care interventions have proven helpful to others in similar situations can aid the care provided by the professional chaplain. A general spiritual pathway around cultural challenge is shown in Figure 1.

In the first step, chaplains identify indicators that may cause spiritual distress for the patient and/or family and conflict with the healthcare staff or the plan of care. This begins by understanding the various components that make up a person's cultural identify. These include the use of symbolic objects; language, patterns of conversation, and tone of voice; non-verbal clues and sense of personal space; concept of time; the structure, composition, and authority of the family or support system; diet, cooking, and dining traditions, and spiritual and religious beliefs and practices. It is helpful when chaplains keep these components in mind as they interact with patients and complete a spiritual assessment.

There are many methods of spiritual assessment. A patient assessment serves to identify and document internal and external resources, spiritual beliefs, important spiritual practices, and the needs and hopes that have arisen during the hospitalization or illness. Often chaplains assist patients in identifying and clarifying these matters. Other items may be included in the spiritual assessment as the chaplain deems appropriate.

Once the assessment is completed and formulated in narrative fashion, the next step, if one utilizes Lucas' "Discipline for Pastoral Care Giving" or a similar tool, is for chaplains to identify what contributing outcomes they hope to provide as a result of interventions. In the case of working with a cultural challenge, one primary contributing outcome would be for the patient to report feeling that the healthcare team respects his or her cultural needs. Note that the emphasis is on respect rather than on understanding. There is always hope that the education provided about any cultural belief or practice will result in better understanding. However, the bottom line issue in patient-centered care is that, whether or not chaplains agree with a belief or practice, they show respect because of its importance to the patient. This is not only a spiritual and emotional need; it is a mandate by the Joint Commission on the Accreditation of Health Care Organizations in its section on patient rights (2003). One way of demonstrating respect is to incorporate that belief or practice into the plan of care in ways that are appropriate in supporting the patient's emotional, physical, and spiritual healing process.

FIGURE 1. Spiritual Pathway for Cultural Challenge Spiritual Issue Addressed: Patient Faces a Healthcare Crisis Outside His/Her Normal Environment

Indicators	Actions/Interventions	Outcomes/Plans
Separation from: • Family • Cultural group • Normal routine, i.e., diet, sleep habits	Establish spiritual care presence Complete spiritual assessment to identify and document patient's: • Internal and external resources including spiritual community • Spiritual Beliefs	Patient identifies spiritual resources and sources of support and is able to utilize them appropriately during hospitalization
Language barrier	• Important spiritual practices • Needs and hopes	Patient reports feeling his/her cultural needs are respected by the healthcare team
Loneliness/isolation/alienation	Assist in activating spiritual resources	Patient reports lessened anxiety
Conflict due to differing expectations and understandings of illness, treatment, and relationship with healthcare team	Identify and document patient's cultural needs and serve as advocate for patient and family	Patient will be able to participate in the environment of care
Seeking meaning in crisis of illness or accident	Provide education for interdisciplinary team as needed regarding identified spiritual and/or cultural needs	Interdisciplinary team will respond to identified issues by adjusting care plan as needed

Other contributing outcomes include assisting patients to: identify their spiritual resources and sources of support as well as ways to utilize them appropriately; experience and report lowered anxiety; and being able to participate in the environment of care. A significant outcome also addresses the chaplains' role as a member of the healthcare team as they provide information and education that leads the interdisciplinary team to adjust the care plan as needed to respond to the identified cultural issues.

Once chaplains know what outcomes they want to contribute, the interventions to bring about those outcomes needs to be named and undertaken. This may include assisting the patient in activating their spiritual resources once they are identified. Or chaplains may need to work in the role of an advocate on behalf of the patient or family with the care team. Perhaps the chaplain may plan a particular religious ritual or find the proper spiritual leaders to do so while negotiating the time and arrangements with the patient's physician, nurse, and other staff. Another intervention might be the sharing of information with a particular interdisciplinary team member about the best way to approach a therapy or intervention and who to include for the intervention to be successful (e.g., a nutritionist who wants to educate a male patient about necessary dietary changes when the patient comes from a traditional patriarchal culture where women do the meal planning and cooking). Or again, chaplains might participate in interdisciplinary team conferences to discuss the patient's plan of care and take a lead role in planning and leading care and decision-making meetings with the patient and/or family.

While it might also be useful to develop pathways for identifiable issues or conflicts that may arise in specific instances–such as the desire of a Native American labor and delivery patient to have the placenta saved for a ritual to be held upon the family's return home–one must take care not to assume a practice is applicable to all patients who appear to share the same culture. To do so would be to practice insensitivity and participate in stereotyping. The intentional focus, rather, raises one's awareness that cultural issues may be present and provides opportunities for conversation in which those issues can be identified and addressed.

Most healthcare professionals prefer the use of clinical language and this is the additional advantage of using the spiritual pathway paradigm. As Lucas (2001) has shown, the role of the chaplain is strengthened and understood more clearly by other members of the team when treatment language is shared.

It is also essential that chaplains document in the patient's chart the cultural issues along with the spiritual and religious ones that arise out of their assessment as well as the identified contributing outcomes and interventions that result. This may call for chaplains to adjust or enhance their current charting practices in order to include a brief description of the cultural practice, its significance and importance to the patient, and the ways in which the practice was or can be preserved, adapted, or repatterned. Conversations with members of the healthcare team are important and cannot be overlooked; however, with the healthcare provider's culture rooted in the habit of charting and utilization of a systematic approach to problem solving, clear and concise documentation is essential.

THE CHAPLAIN AS EDUCATOR
CONCERNING CULTURAL SENSITIVITY

Both medical and nursing educators are finding themselves currently in the midst of a major paradigm shift from structure-and process-based to competency-based education. It is important that professional chaplains know what this change in educational focus is and what its impact is upon the healthcare environment. Competency-based education focuses and functions by defining the desired outcomes of the training (Carraccio, 2002). "Competency" within this model is defined as "a complex set of behaviors built on the components of knowledge, skills, attitudes, and personal ability." In addition, those who advocate for this change also highlight the critical importance of planning to identify and define the specific competencies needed for professional practice (del Bueno, 1986). The focus is on benchmarking performance indicators in order to describe and achieve expected outcomes for each competency (Lemons, 1998). The knowledge, skills, and attitudes underpinning each competency are to be clearly written and measurable.

Within the arena of cultural competence, healthcare workers are required to develop many behaviors. To understand how challenging this endeavor is, one must understand the dynamics involved in developing education resources and the teaching of healthcare professionals. One must have a strong background in adult learning theory and teaching techniques and realize that nurses, physicians, and other clinical staff have unique approaches to and expectations for their learning. A general rule of thumb is that while many individuals enjoy the theoretical part of learning concepts and theories, most healthcare professionals are more interested in-and tune into-what impact the learning has upon their clinical practice. Knowledge of cultural, spiritual, and religious differences is important; for the healthcare professional what is even more important is how to use that knowledge in clear and concrete ways in the course of one's work. The White Paper (VandeCreek and Burton, 2001) highlights the role of the professional chaplain as an educator for the healthcare team whose role is "interpreting and analyzing multi-faith and multi-cultural traditions as they impact clinical services." Chaplains who are currently incorporating teaching opportunities into their daily interactions with clinical staff as well as those who want to begin doing so, need to pay attention to these learning needs. One way in which professional chaplaincy groups can support this is by providing the resources necessary for chaplains to gain the tools that they need to be successful and effective educators.

Where do professional chaplains teach about cultural and spiritual sensitivity issues? Formal classes can be held as a part of new clinical employee orientation, as a part of a medical education program for new resident orientation or grand rounds, or as a presentation done at a nursing, medical, or other professional workshop. Informal teaching is done during interdisciplinary rounds, unit-based meetings, and in the multitude of conversations that chaplains have with nurses, physicians, therapists, and other members of the team. Chaplains who participated in the beta study of Wintz and Cooper (2000) showed numerous creative ways in which they utilized the materials within their organizations; in all of them the chaplain functioned as educator, advocate, and resource.

CONCLUSION

Fukuyama and Sevig raise the important question concerning how cultural diversity impacts the work of health care chaplains. Here I emphasize that chaplains be aware of how they are a professional resource for the practice of cultural and spiritual sensitivity within healthcare organizations. By nature of their unique role and scope of practice, professional chaplains walk with patients and families during health events that more often than not impact them in life-changing ways. Practicing cultural and spiritual sensitivity and educating others within one's organization about its importance is a natural part of the chaplain's work. As professional members of the healthcare team, chaplains are called to respond to this challenge. May we do so with enthusiasm, creativity, and dedication!

AUTHOR NOTE

Sue Wintz has provided professional ministry for over 25 years as a congregational pastor and a board certified professional chaplain in both community hospitals and urban medical centers. She is a Presbyterian (USA) Minister of Word and Sacrament. During the past ten years, she has increased her appreciation for cultural differences and for spiritual sensitivity, providing ministry in a Arizona-Mexico border community and within Phoenix, Arizona. She currently teaches cultural and spiritual sensitivity within the medical center for clinical staff, medical residents, Clinical Pastoral Education programs, and professional healthcare groups. Under her leadership, the chaplaincy department functions as the "cultural brokers" within the institution, putting into practice the skills and expertise outlined in this article.

REFERENCES

Carraccio, C. (2002) "Shifting paradigms: From Flexner to competencies." *Academic Medicine*. 17:5, 361-367.
del Bueno, D.J. (1986) "Competency based education." *Nurse Educator*. 3:10-14.
Hilsman, G. (1998) "A spiritual pathway for prior grief." *Chaplaincy Today*. 14:2.

Joint Commission for the Accreditation of Healthcare Organizations. 2003. *Comprehensive Accreditation Manual for Hospitals.* Oakbrook Terrace, IL. www.jcaho.org.

Lemons, D.E., and Grisold, J.G. (1998) "Defining the Boundaries of Physiological Understanding: The Benchmarks Curriculum Model." *Advanced Physiological Education.* 20:S35-245.

Lucas, A. and VandeCreek L. (2001) *The Discipline for Pastoral Care Giving.* Binghamton, NY. The Haworth Press, Inc.

VandeCreek, L. and Burton, L. (2001) *Professional Chaplaincy: Its Role and Importance in Healthcare: A White Paper.* Shaumburg, IL. Association of Professional Chaplains.

Wintz, S. and Cooper, E. (2000). *Learning Model for Cultural and Spiritual Sensitivity* and *Quick Guides to Cultures and Traditions. www.professionalchaplains.org*

Wintz, S. and Cooper E. (2003) "Developing Learning Materials to Address Cultural and Spiritual Sensitivity." *Chaplaincy Today;* 19:2.

Index

BOOK ORDER FORM!

Order a copy of this book with this form or online at:
http://www.haworthpress.com/store/product.asp?sku=5247

Ministry in the Spiritual and Cultural Diversity of Health Care
Increasing the Competency of Chaplains

____ in softbound at $19.95 (ISBN: 0-7890-2557-4)
____ in hardbound at $29.95 (ISBN: 0-7890-2556-6)

COST OF BOOKS _____

POSTAGE & HANDLING _____
US: $4.00 for first book & $1.50
for each additional book
Outside US: $5.00 for first book
& $2.00 for each additional book.

SUBTOTAL _____

In Canada: add 7% GST. _____

STATE TAX _____
CA, IL, IN, MN, NJ, NY, OH & SD residents
please add appropriate local sales tax.

FINAL TOTAL _____
If paying in Canadian funds, convert
using the current exchange rate,
UNESCO coupons welcome.

❏ BILL ME LATER:
Bill-me option is good on US/Canada/
Mexico orders only; not good to jobbers,
wholesalers, or subscription agencies.

❏ Signature _____

❏ Payment Enclosed: $ _____

❏ PLEASE CHARGE TO MY CREDIT CARD:
❏ Visa ❏ MasterCard ❏ AmEx ❏ Discover
❏ Diner's Club ❏ Eurocard ❏ JCB

Account # _____

Exp Date _____

Signature _____
(Prices in US dollars and subject to change without notice.)

PLEASE PRINT ALL INFORMATION OR ATTACH YOUR BUSINESS CARD

Name

Address

City   State/Province   Zip/Postal Code

Country

Tel   Fax

E-Mail

May we use your e-mail address for confirmations and other types of information? ❏ Yes ❏ No We appreciate receiving
your e-mail address. Haworth would like to e-mail special discount offers to you, as a preferred customer.
We will never share, rent, or exchange your e-mail address. We regard such actions as an invasion of your privacy.

Order From Your **Local Bookstore** or Directly From
The Haworth Press, Inc. 10 Alice Street, Binghamton, New York 13904-1580 • USA
Call Our toll-free number (1-800-429-6784) / Outside US/Canada: (607) 722-5857
Fax: 1-800-895-0582 / Outside US/Canada: (607) 771-0012
E-mail your order to us: orders@haworthpress.com

For orders outside US and Canada, you may wish to order through your local
sales representative, distributor, or bookseller.
For information, see http://haworthpress.com/distributors

(Discounts are available for individual orders in US and Canada only, not booksellers/distributors.)

Please photocopy this form for your personal use.
www.HaworthPress.com

BOF04

LINCOLN CHRISTIAN UNIVERSITY